THE PEDIATRICIAN'S
GUIDE TO
FEEDING
BABIES
& TODDLERS

THE PEDIATRICIAN'S
GUIDE TO
FEEDING
BABIES
& TODDLERS

Practical Answers to Your
Questions on Nutrition,
Starting Solids, Allergies,
Picky Eating, and More

ANTHONY F. PORTO, MD MPH
DINA M. DIMAGGIO, MD

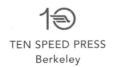

TEN SPEED PRESS
Berkeley

CONTENTS

Dedication

We dedicate this book to our inspirations, our children, Julia, Evie, Sebby, Sid, Annie, Aaron, Sean, Andi, Jolie, Azriel, Anna, Emilia, and Caleb, and also to all the children we have been fortunate enough to take care of over the years; we cannot express enough how grateful we are to be allowed into your lives.

Introduction

The Pediatrician's Guide to Feeding Babies & Toddlers combines the expertise of a group of pediatricians, a dietitian, a lactation consultant, and two chefs. More importantly, we are also parents to a total of thirteen children. Most of us met during our medical training and cultivated strong friendships during our long days and nights working together in a hospital. After completing our training over a decade ago, we felt that we were prepared to practice medicine. We couldn't imagine, however, how much our careers would be enhanced by our roles as parents. When Dina's daughters, Julia and Evelyn, were born just twenty-one months apart, Dina realized she didn't really know how a mother was feeling until she was a mother herself. As we were writing this book, Anthony was learning the ins and outs of fatherhood as he cared for his newborn son, Sebastian. Persephone was busy chasing after her twin toddler boys, Sean and Aaron. Janet bonded with her newborn daughter, Annie, and toddler son, Sid. Liza was busy helping her daughters, Emilia and Anna, with their homework and coordinating after-school activities; Susan was going on college tours with her son, Caleb; Alison developed recipes while tending to her newborn son, Azriel; and Dini cooked alongside her little girl, Andi, while taking care of her newborn daughter, Jolie. Caring for our own children helped us understand the fears, anxieties, and questions of parents on a deeper level.

Over the years, we have discussed how often parents would ask the same questions about feeding their children. We found that parents did not know where to turn for guidance and became frustrated with trying to find the right information on their own. We also know that Google-searching (yes, we all do this, often in the middle of the night!) can lead to anxiety and confusion.

We believe that feeding should be fun, stress-free, and family-oriented quality time. We created this book as a resource to provide easy access to common feeding questions from the minute an infant is born through the toddler years.

Dina, a general pediatrician, and Anthony, a pediatric gastroenterologist, who are the lead authors, assembled a team that includes a pediatric allergist, a developmental-behavioral pediatrician, a pediatric dietitian, and a lactation consultant, along with two family chefs to help answer common feeding and nutrition questions. This book was also reviewed for completeness and accuracy by an additional board-certified general pediatrician. The goal is to present the most current evidence-based information in an easy-to-read question-and-answer format. We understand the reality of parenthood and use this knowledge, along with our medical acumen, to develop practical approaches to the feeding and care of infants and toddlers. We want the best beginnings for the children we take care of, for our own children, and for your children.

How to Use This Book

We have divided the book into five age groups from the newborn period to the early toddler years. Every section contains expected developmental milestones, basic nutritional guidelines, expected growth, common medical concerns, and ends with developmentally appropriate recipes for that stage.

In chapter one, we discuss infants from birth to 3 months of life and end with healthy recipes for hungry caregivers. In chapter two, the 4 to 6 months group, we discuss the new challenge of how best to feed a baby solid foods. In chapters three and four, we discuss the 7 to 8 month and 9 to 12 month age groups, respectively. As your child increases intake of solid foods, we will address common questions such as balancing solid food and milk intake and how to transition to finger foods. In chapter five, we focus on the early toddler years, guiding parents on how to deal with picky eaters and providing healthy choices as children enter the school years. We end with chapter six, which discusses the most common medical concerns in more detail and includes additional resources.

We designed this book not only to be a reference, but also a reassuring guide through the stage that your baby is in or about to go through. You can, therefore, use this book in multiple ways—by quickly finding out the answer to a current concern, by reading the section that your baby is in now or about to be in, by reading the entire book and then referring back to particular sections later as you need them, or by referencing chapter six to find out more details about a specific medical concern.

We look forward to sharing our knowledge about infant and toddler nutrition, learned from our many collective years of caring for children in the medical field, combined with our practical experiences as parents ourselves. Raising a child provides you with some of the most extraordinary times in your life, but as we know, it can also be stressful. We hope to ease this journey by providing you with information you can trust and valuable insights into the world of childhood nutrition, so you can spend less time searching for answers and more time enjoying these fleeting moments.

Chapter One

~~~~~~~~~~~~~~~~

0 to 3 Months

In chapter one, we discuss infants from birth to 3 months of life. Newborns bring overwhelming joy but also a great sense of responsibility. When your baby is only a few days old and comes to his/her first doctor's appointment, all the fears that overwhelm sleep-deprived new parents come to the surface: Is my baby eating enough? Is his/her poop the right color? Is my baby gaining enough weight? How do I store breast milk or formula? Am I producing enough breast milk or using the best formula? In this section, we guide you with answers to all of these questions. We will also discuss common medical issues including milk allergies, acid reflux, and constipation. We end with healthy recipes for breastfeeding moms and hungry parents.

Expected Developmental Milestones

In the first few days of life, your baby will do a whole lot of sleeping, eating, wetting and soiling diapers, passing gas, fussing and crying, and not a whole lot more. Although children will meet their developmental milestones on their own time line, we have listed below some of the milestones you can look forward to at the ages in this section, and will also list the expected milestones for other stages throughout this book. We hope they will help you understand how feeding and nourishment are related to development and a baby's ability to feed. If you are concerned about your child's development, talk to your pediatrician. You can also read about physical developmental delays at motordelay.aap.org.

By 1 month, a baby's gross motor skills should include raising the head slightly when on his/her tummy and moving the head from side to side. Visually they can see eight to twelve inches away, focus, track light and objects with their eyes (but may be cross-eyed), and can follow objects moved in front of them to the middle of their face, but usually not a full 180 degrees. Even as newborns, babies have a visual preference for the human face. Babies can hear well and will startle easily. Socially, they prefer soft touch, and if breastfeeding, the scent of their mother's breast milk. Crying peaks at 6 weeks of age at which time infants may cry for three hours per day. By 12 weeks of age, infants typically cry for one hour per day.

Colic

Colic, a common condition in the newborn period, starts around 2 to 3 weeks, peaks at 6 to 8 weeks, and usually resolves around 3 or 4 months. It is associated with fussiness and crying for three or more hours a day, three or more days per week, and can make feeding difficult. Babies will have periods of crying that will typically begin in the evening hours (you may hear it referred to as the "witching" hours) and last until the wee hours of the morning. The episodes of crying associated with colic are intense, and babies sound distressed and tend to start and stop suddenly. There is no definite known cause or treatment for colic, but most parents believe their baby is gassy or suffering from indigestion during this time. The good news is that it will pass in a few short (or long) weeks. Since colic may often be stressful for new parents, support from other parents who also have colicky babies or from your baby's pediatrician may be helpful during this phase.

Developmental Milestones from Birth to 3 Months

AGE	MOTOR AND VISUAL SKILLS	SOCIAL SKILLS	COGNITIVE/ LANGUAGE
1 month	Startles, raises head while on tummy, moves head from side to side, hands are in fisted position, can follow objects moved in front of them to midline, focuses 8 to 12 inches, eyes may cross.	Prefers soft touch rather than rough handling, likes sweet smells and if breastfeeding, prefers the scent of their mother's breast milk, may have fussiness or colicky periods.	Can hear well and may turn to sounds, likes to look at black-and-white pictures and especially at faces, expresses needs with crying.
2 months	Will lift up head more when on belly and may lift chest off ground, fists are not clenched as tightly, visually, eyes are more coordinated, will follow objects past the midline or a full 180 degrees and will see further distances.	Develops a social smile, recognizes parents.	Starts to make vowel sounds.
3 months	Able to lift up on chest more during tummy time and hold head up steadily, opens and closes fists, stares at hands, brings hands to mouth, begins to swat at objects.	Recognizes familiar people and rewards them with a smile or reaches toward them, starts to imitate some facial expressions.	Coos.

Adapted from The Harriet Lane Handbook, *17 Edition, and* AAP Caring for Your Baby and Young Child, Birth to Age 5, *4th Edition.*

FEEDING SKILLS

Able to suck/swallow liquids. Has the rooting reflex—when lips/cheek are stroked, mouth will turn toward the object allowing baby to turn toward food. Tongue thrust or extrusion reflex causes a baby's tongue to move out when the lips are touched, which aids in breast or bottle feeding.

At 2 months, gross motor skills include lifting up their heads and chests more when they are on their bellies. Visually, they will follow objects past the midline or a full 180 degrees. Socially, babies will make some vowel sounds, will develop a social smile, and will recognize their parents, making those sleepless nights well worth it. Infants may also sleep longer, often four to nine hour stretches at night.

At 3 months, more of a routine has developed and your infant will likely change dramatically into a playful, interactive baby! Gross motor skills include lifting their chests off the ground, opening and closing their fists, swatting at objects, staring at their hands, and bringing their hands to their mouth. They often begin a stage where they drool throughout the day (teeth might come out weeks to months later, although they usually appear between 4 to 12 months old). Socially, a 3-month-old will recognize familiar people and reward them with a smile, and will start to imitate some facial expressions and coo.

Basic Nutritional Guidelines

Since babies don't come with any instructions, it may be difficult for parents to determine the best ways to support their growing infants. This section guides parents on how to know if your baby is hungry or full, if he/she is getting enough to eat, and if your baby needs any supplements at this stage. These insights will help allay anxieties as you get to know your baby's feeding patterns.

How much and how often will my child eat?

First, a little math. Mostly you will need to know ounces and milliliters (mL). This will give you an idea of how small your child's stomach is, and will help you make feeding decisions (see chart opposite).

The amount your baby may drink will vary and some babies will take more at one feeding and less at another. If your baby shows signs of wanting more formula, gradually increase the amount your baby is receiving; for example, try offering an additional half of an ounce. If it is refused, don't force it, but if your baby wants more, give more. Likewise, if your baby seems hungry prior to the expected time of breastfeeding, he/she may be ready for a feeding sooner than expected, and it is okay to offer the breast or additional expressed breast milk. The table "Average Ounces of Formula Per Day and How Often to Breastfeed" on page 6 should give you an idea about how much babies usually take at each stage. This guide provides approximations only, and it is okay if your baby drinks different amounts, at different frequencies. The best rule is to simply follow his/her cues rather than a fixed amount. During the first two weeks of life, formula-fed infants may actually eat less. This decrease is normal as long as they remain hydrated and have approximately six wet diapers daily after one week of life, stool regularly (some babies stool with each feeding, others can skip a few days), and are gaining weight. They will gradually increase the volume of each feeding, and eventually, both formula- and breastfed-infants will be on a more consistent feeding pattern of every three to four hours during the day.

When I'm asked how often my baby feeds, what exactly does that mean?
You can determine the time between feedings from the *start* of one feeding to the *start* of the next feeding. For example, if your baby starts feeding at 10:00 a.m., and begins to feed again at 1:00 p.m. and at 4:00 p.m., your baby is feeding every three hours.

How do I know if my baby is hungry or full?
During the first few weeks, babies will feed on demand, about every two to three hours for breastfeeding babies and every three to four hours for formula-fed babies during the daytime. Babies may go longer stretches at nighttime. Your infants

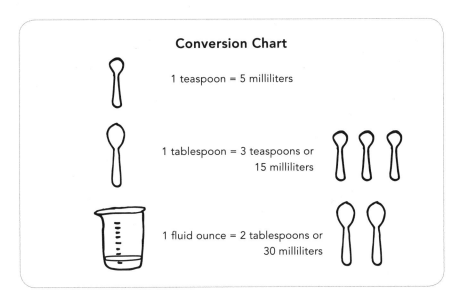

Conversion Chart

1 teaspoon = 5 milliliters

1 tablespoon = 3 teaspoons or 15 milliliters

1 fluid ounce = 2 tablespoons or 30 milliliters

Size of a Child's Stomach

Day 1	5–7 mL	about 1 teaspoon
Day 2	22–27 mL	about 1 ounce
Day 3	45–60 mL	about 1½–2 ounces
Adult	900 mL	2 cups

Adapted from Dunham's Premature Infants, *3rd Edition.*

Average Ounces of Formula Per Day and How Often to Breastfeed

AGE	AVERAGE OUNCES OF FORMULA	HOW OFTEN TO BREASTFEED
Full-term newborn	2 ounces per bottle approximately every 3–4 hours	On demand, approximately every 2–3 hours, or 8–12 times per day
1 month	3–4 ounces per bottle every 3–4 hours	On demand, approximately every 2–4 hours, or 7–8 times per day
2–4 months	3–6 ounces per bottle, 5–8 times per day	On demand, approximately 5–8 times per day
4–6 months	4–6 ounces per bottle, 4–6 times per day	4–6 times per day
6–8 months	6–8 ounces per bottle, 3–5 times per day	3–5 times per day
8–12 months	7–8 ounces per bottle, 3–4 times per day	3–4 times per day
12 months and up	Approximately 16 to a maximum of 24 ounces of whole milk per day (formula can be changed to whole milk at 1 year)	Is individually based from 1 to 2 times to multiple times per day

Adapted from USDA Food and Nutrition Service's Infant Nutrition and Feeding Guide for Use in the WIC and CSF Programs and Texas Children's Hospital Pediatric Reference Guide.

will let you know if they are hungry by opening their mouths, making sucking sounds, smacking their lips, bobbing their heads up and down across your chest, rooting (turning their cheek to the side that is stroked), sucking on their hands and fingers, and becoming more alert and fussy. Crying is a late hunger sign and you will soon learn your baby's hunger cues before crying begins. When they are full, babies will fall asleep at the breast or bottle, turn away from the nipple, or slow down and stop sucking.

Should I worry if my baby loses weight right after birth? How do I know if my child is getting enough breast milk or formula?

It is normal for babies to lose some weight in the first days of life. Monitor your newborn's urine output as this will be a rough indicator that your baby is getting enough fluid (See "Normal Urine Output for a newborn" on page 8). If your infant seems unsatisfied after feeding, is consistently crying despite being comforted and fed on cue, is feeding so frequently you cannot tell one feeding from the next, or is feeding for hours on end, your baby may not be getting enough milk. If your baby is showing any signs of dehydration (See table "Common Signs of Dehydration" on page 8), you should contact your pediatrician. Signs that your newborn may not be gaining weight appropriately are also if your newborn loses ten percent or more of his/her birth weight or has not returned to birth weight by the second or third week of life.

Your pediatrician or a lactation consultant along with your pediatrician, if you are breastfeeding, will help you come up with the best strategies to ensure your baby is growing appropriately for his/her age. If your child is not gaining weight appropriately, they may suggest ways to help increase your milk

Range of Calories per Day

AGE	CALORIES PER DAY*
1–3 Months	Males: 472–572
	Females: 438–521

*This range of calories is an estimate based on the average child. Your child may require more or less calories.

Adapted from USDA Food and Nutrition Service's Infant Nutrition and Feeding Guide for Use in the WIC and CSF Programs.

supply and may ask you to supplement with formula or expressed breast milk. If your child is formula feeding, your doctor may discuss ways to increase your infant's calorie intake. They may also have your baby come in for more frequent weight checks.

Remember, it is not uncommon for some babies to gain weight slowly at first, but with a little guidance, babies will catch up and will start gaining weight appropriately or an average a half an ounce to an ounce a day.

Normal Urine Output for a Newborn Infant

DAYS OF LIFE	NUMBER OF WET DIAPERS PER DAY
1 day	1+ wet diaper
2 days	2+ wet diapers
3 days	3+ wet diapers
1 week or when mother's milk is fully in	6+ wet diapers

Common Signs of Dehydration

Decrease in the number of wet diapers

Urine dark yellow and concentrated or urate crystals (salmon colored spots in diaper) present*

Anterior fontanel (soft spot on the top of the head) sunken in

Overly sleepy or irritable

*If you are concerned about discoloration found in your baby's diaper, you should bring it to your pediatrician's attention. If you find clear crystals that resemble kosher salt, however, it might be from a ripped or damaged diaper. The "salt" is from the inside of the diaper leaking out—cut a diaper open and see for yourself!

Do I need to give my newborn any supplements?

Although breast milk provides the majority of the nutrients your baby needs, it does not provide enough vitamin D for growing babies. Vitamin D is important for bone growth. Our body produces vitamin D when our skin is exposed to direct sunlight. Small babies are kept out of direct sunlight and are covered in sunscreen after 6 months old, when sunscreen is approved for use in babies. These practices block vitamin D production. Rickets, a rare condition caused by severe vitamin D deficiency, can occur if a baby isn't receiving adequate vitamin D and has limited sunlight exposure (it may be surprising to see such vitamin deficiencies in our modern society, but we have occasionally seen these conditions in our medical practices). New research suggests that maternal vitamin D supplementation with 6400 IU per day results in adequate vitamin D levels in the exclusively breastfed baby. However, this information is still new and currently supplementing mothers with very high amounts of vitamin D is *not* standard of care. Therefore, all exclusively breast fed babies should be supplemented with 400 IU (International Units) of vitamin D each day starting at a few days old. Babies should continue taking vitamin D throughout the first year of breastfeeding, or if weaned or partially breastfed, until they are consuming thirty-two ounces of formula or are transitioned to vitamin D–fortified whole milk at a year of age. Likewise, if exclusively formula-fed babies are consuming less than thirty-two ounces of formula a day, they may also need a vitamin D supplement. We recommend talking to your pediatrician about what they recommend is best for your baby.

Vitamin supplements can be found over the counter at most pharmacies. Some popular brands are Tri-Vi-Sol, which contains vitamins A, C, and D; D-Vi-Sol, which solely contains vitamin D; and Carlson vitamin D drops, which contain vitamin D and E. Carlson drops may be easier to administer, since one drop contains the daily recommended 400 IU of vitamin D, while other brands require 1 mL to reach the same dose. We recommend carefully following the manufacturer's directions and pediatrician's instructions for dosing and dropping the vitamin on your baby's inner cheek or placing it on your nipple for your baby to drink. If your baby is drinking from a bottle, you can also try adding the vitamin to the bottle.

Other supplements parents often ask about are multivitamins, iron, and fluoride. If your baby was born prematurely or was found to be anemic, your pediatrician may recommend a multivitamin or iron supplement. These supplements are usually unnecessary in healthy full-term infants.

Fluoride supplements are not needed during the first six months of life. These may be necessary after 6 months of age until 16 years of life if your drinking water contains less than 0.3 parts per million of fluoride to ensure dental health. Formulas contain minimal fluoride whether in powdered, concentrated, or ready-to-feed forms, but fluoride can come from the tap water you use when you're preparing a bottle, if using a concentrated or powdered formula. You should discuss with your pediatrician the need for fluoride supplementation.

Vitamin D, Iron, and Fluoride

Vitamin D maintains normal calcium and phosphorus levels in the body by helping the body to absorb them from the diet. Calcium and phosphorus are needed to maintain healthy bones. Factors that decrease the amount of vitamin D that your body can make include decreased sun exposure, especially due to the use of sunscreen, living in areas with higher air pollution or in areas with dense clouds blocking sunlight. Darker-skinned individuals are also more at risk for vitamin D deficiency. Severe vitamin D deficiency may lead to rickets and weaker bones.

Iron is a mineral that serves many functions in our bodies. One of its main functions is to help produce red blood cells and to transport oxygen throughout our body. See page 135 for more information about iron and iron-deficiency anemia.

Fluoride is a mineral that helps prevent tooth decay and promotes good dental health. Fluoride helps to harden the enamel of teeth and helps protect teeth from acid damage that occurs while eating, when sugars combine with bacteria present in our mouths.

Feeding Options

The baby has finally arrived! Now the next big question is "How do you plan on feeding your infant"? The main methods of feeding a baby are by breastfeeding, giving expressed breast milk, formula feeding, or a combination of these methods. As pediatricians, we believe the optimal way to feed your baby is by the method that works best for you, your family, and your baby (and not the way your neighbor or popular blog says is best). What matters most to us is that your baby is in a loving environment, and that your baby is growing well and is happy and healthy, albeit from breast milk, formula, or breast milk with formula supplementation.

Breastfeeding

Breastfeeding will provide your baby with all the nutrients needed to grow and develop. The benefits of breastfeeding are well documented and the American Academy of Pediatrics (or AAP, a professional organization of pediatricians that guides health care standards in children) recommends exclusive breastfeeding for approximately six months, after which breastfeeding is continued, along with complementary foods, until the baby is 1 year old or for as long as mom desires to breastfeed. Some of the potential benefits of breastfeeding include a reduction in upper respiratory and gastrointestinal infections, a reduction in ear infections, bronchiolitis, obesity, and type one diabetes. Breastfeeding is also beneficial to mothers—it may reduce the risks of high blood pressure, heart disease, type two diabetes, breast and ovarian cancer, and helps many moms return to their prepregnancy weight.

For many lucky mothers, when their baby is first born and placed on the breast, the baby latches with ease, and it is smooth sailing from the very beginning. For other mothers, not so much. When mothers struggle with sore nipples, difficulty latching, and low milk supply, the frustration is often accompanied by a roller coaster of emotions. We highly encourage new parents to get support from family, friends, new parent groups, and to seek advice from a lactation consultant, pediatrician, or other health care professional if they need help with breastfeeding. Breastfeeding can take time to get the hang of, but with appropriate help and a little patience, these difficulties usually resolve. With that said, some mothers choose not to breastfeed and other parents are not able to. We all too often encounter a teary mother whose breastfeeding is not going as smoothly as planned. She is hard on herself and feels guilty about giving her baby supplemental formula or a bottle with expressed breast milk. Again, we ultimately recommend what is best for both the parent or parents and the child. Once breastfeeding is established, feeding your baby a bottle with expressed breast milk or formula does not often interfere with the baby taking the breast later on. If your goal is to feed your baby as much of mom's own milk as possible, a board-certified lactation consultant can often advise you on how to take those breaks without sacrificing milk supply. Breastfeeding is hard work, and raising a newborn is even harder, so take a break and rest when you need it!

What is known about breastfeeding and development of childhood allergies?

Here is a summary of what is known about the benefits of exclusive breastfeeding on the development of childhood allergic diseases:

- Exclusive breastfeeding for three to four months reduces the number of episodes of early respiratory viral-induced wheezing before age 4.
- Exclusive breastfeeding for four to six months may reduce the incidence of atopic dermatitis (eczema) for children before age 2.
- Exclusive breastfeeding may also reduce the incidence of cow's milk allergy (but not all food allergies) before age 2.

- It is not clear whether exclusive breastfeeding has an effect on the development of allergic rhinitis (an allergic reaction to allergens you breath in, more commonly called hay fever), other food allergies, later childhood asthma, or eczema after age 2.

Should I avoid certain foods while breastfeeding to prevent allergies in my baby?

The short answer to this frequently asked question is no. We have talked to hundreds of mothers of food-allergic children who question whether there was something they ate or did during pregnancy, or while breastfeeding, that could have either caused or prevented their child's food allergy. For instance, mothers often wonder if they should avoid eating peanuts to prevent their child from developing a peanut allergy.

At this point, large studies have *not* shown any allergy-preventative benefits from altering nursing mothers' diets. The allergy experts who reviewed all

Real Life Parenting

When Janet had her first child, Sid, she expected breastfeeding to be easy and come naturally. Sid, however, had a difficult time latching; Janet's milk was slow to come in; and Sid was jaundiced. At the recommendation of her pediatrician, she gave formula while she attempted to breastfeed and then reached out for support from a lactation consultant. She was at first disappointed and almost embarrassed to be a dietician who wouldn't be able to exclusively breastfeed, but later came to realize that a healthy, well-nourished baby is much more important than an expectation of how she imagined breastfeeding would be.

Dina also thought that because she was a pediatrician who advocated for breastfeeding on a routine basis, that as soon as her daughter was born she was going to absolutely love breastfeeding and would immediately be able to breastfeed with great ease. This could be the case for many, but not for Dina. Breastfeeding hurt. She was emotional, tired, and felt guilty that she was having thoughts of quitting. With the help of nurses and lactation consultants at NYU Medical Center, it did get easier and more enjoyable. Although many new moms might feel like they are the only one having difficulty with feeding, they are absolutely not alone!

published studies to come up with the national food allergy practice guidelines (updated in 2014) did not find evidence that maternal allergen avoidance prevented allergic diseases in breastfeeding infants. In addition, a study reviewing five major clinical trials that looked at whether maternal dietary restrictions could affect eczema in breastfeeding babies concluded that there was no evidence to suggest that avoidance of allergenic foods during lactation had any impact on preventing eczema in the first one and a half years of a child's life.

This is an involved answer to this fairly simple question, we know, but this does show that this is a hot issue in the pediatric allergy world. Although we don't think that there is any reason to avoid allergenic foods (like peanuts, milk, wheat, or eggs) while you are nursing your baby, it is possible that results of research that is going on now may someday change our minds and thus our recommendations.

What are the different stages of breast milk? When will my milk come in and how will I know?

The first milk your breasts will produce is colostrum, which can be clear or yellowish and creamy in color. Colostrum is packed full of nutrients, antibodies, and protein. It is low in fat, easily digestible, and should be all your baby needs in the first few days. Colostrum also helps a baby to pass his/her first sticky black stool, or meconium.

You will know your milk is in when your breasts start to feel harder or engorged, milk leaks, and the color of the thicker colostrum changes to transitional milk. This transitional milk, which usually is produced two to five days after giving birth, contains high levels of fat, sugar (lactose), and more calories than colostrum. You may also experience a milk letdown or milk ejection reflex (a tingling feeling) which occurs when milk is pushed out of your milk producing cells into milk ducts, releasing the breast milk for feeding. The letdown is usually triggered by nursing, pumping, or by the sound of your crying baby. When your baby is around 10 to 15 days old, transitional milk turns into mature milk, which is composed of foremilk (the milk at the start of the feeding) and hindmilk (the breast milk at the end of the feeding). Your milk may look more watery in appearance at the beginning of the feeding when your milk has higher levels of water, lactose, vitamins, and proteins (foremilk) and creamier near the end of the feeding (hindmilk) as the levels of fat rise. Over the course of twenty-four hours, most babies will get an adequate mixture of all the components of breast milk regardless of how thin or thick your milk looks at a particular feeding. Sometimes pumping large quantities of extra milk after feeding your baby on the breast may create an imbalance if you are storing more of the fatty part of the milk in the freezer than is being fed to your baby. If your baby is fussy, you may need to cut back on stocking the freezer.

Is there anything I can take that will increase my milk supply?

Many breastfeeding mothers may try different herbal or nutritional supplements or foods to help increase their milk supply. Unfortunately, there is no one "it" food or supplement a new mother can take to increase her milk supply, and even the more common supplements the American Academy of Pediatrics (AAP) generally recognizes as safe, such as fenugreek, may occasionally result in side effects such as low blood sugar and dizziness. Before taking any supplement, we recommend that mothers talk to their obstetrician or midwife to determine if it is right for them and to seek the help of a lactation consultant or other health care professional for suggestions on how to troubleshoot milk supply problems.

How long can I store my breast milk?

According to La Leche League International, breast milk for healthy full-term infants can be stored at room temperature (66 to 78°F) for four hours, in a refrigerator (lower than 39°F) for three days, and in a freezer (0°F) of a refrigerator with separate doors for three to six months. The Centers for Disease Control and Prevention (CDC) and the Academy of Breastfeeding Medicine recommend longer storage times, and suggest storing breast milk at room temperature for up to six to eight hours, in the refrigerator for up to five days, and the freezer compartment of the refrigerator with separate doors for three to six months. If you want to make life simple, follow a more conservative approach by using the "rule of threes"—three hours at room temperature, three days in the refrigerator, and three months in the freezer. It is preferred that milk be stored in the back of the refrigerator or freezer, where it is coldest and not affected as much by temperature variations with opening and closing of doors. And when in doubt,

Rule of Threes for Breast Milk Storage for Full-Term Infants

- **3 hours** at room temperature
- **3 days** in the refrigerator
- **3 months** in the freezer

do like you do when you add milk to your morning cereal—smell it! If it smells bad, it probably is bad, and needs to be discarded.

How do I thaw and warm breast milk? Can I reuse it later?

The best way to thaw frozen breast milk is in a refrigerator overnight, by holding it under warm water from a faucet, or by placing it in a bowl of warm water. Don't be surprised if your breast milk separates into two layers, a fatty layer on top and a watery layer on the bottom. You simply need to shake the bottle gently so that the layers mix prior to feeding. Once thawed, breast milk should not be refrozen, should be stored in a refrigerator, and should be consumed within twenty-four hours.

To warm breast milk from the refrigerator, you can place the bottle in a bowl of warm water or run it under warm water. A bottle warmer is convenient but not necessary. We always recommend squirting a few drops of milk onto the back of your hand to double check that the temperature is lukewarm before feeding it to your baby. You should never warm bottles in the microwave, as microwaves unevenly heat the milk and the milk can then burn your baby's mouth. Microwaves can also affect the constituents of breast milk. Placing a bottle of milk directly in water that is boiling on the stove or heating it directly on the stove should also be avoided, again to prevent the baby from getting burned from milk that is too hot and to prevent damaging the nutrients found in breast milk.

Even though breast milk is supposed to have antibacterial factors, the research on the topic of what happens when saliva gets into the milk is not yet clear. We would be cautious and recommend discarding the residual breast milk that is left after a baby drinks from the bottle and not saving the breast milk for later use. If you do decide to give your baby leftover breast milk from a previous bottle, we recommend keeping it for no more than the next feeding and always smelling or tasting it prior to feeding it to your baby. Try not to overfill your baby's bottle beyond what your baby typically drinks so you can spend less time pondering whether to save or toss leftover milk. This also helps remove the temptation to encourage your baby to take more than he/she wants because you don't want to toss that precious milk leftover in the bottle. You can start off by offering two ounces of breast milk at a time and can always add more milk into your baby's bottle if your baby is hungrier.

Can I use a pacifier if my baby is fussy, or will this create nipple confusion?

This is a hot topic! Parents are often made to be fearful of pacifiers and are told that once the pacifier hits a baby's mouth, the baby will forget how to breastfeed.

Pacifier Weaning

The American Academy of Family Physicians (AAFP) and the AAP recommend weaning pacifiers after 6 months old to reduce the chances of babies getting ear infections and later dental issues. The longer caregivers wait to remove the pacifier, the harder it will be, since pacifiers often become a beloved source of comfort. For younger infants, it is easiest to go cold turkey. For older children, you can try a gradual wean by only allowing the pacifier while napping or at bedtime and then taking it away completely, by giving it away in exchange for a new toy or object of comfort, or by giving it as a present to a younger baby.

The hospitals that participate in the Baby Friendly Hospital Initiative are particularly strict in that they do not allow pacifiers on the postpartum floor. Where do we stand? We are not opposed to the use of pacifiers. Babies often like to suck to help sooth themselves. If you are choosing to nurse, once breastfeeding is well established and your baby is gaining weight appropriately, it is completely fine to offer a pacifier. Likewise, babies fed expressed breast milk or formula may also use a pacifier for comfort. In fact, the AAP states that you should consider using a pacifier when breastfeeding is established at 3 to 4 weeks, at sleep time and naps, as there is evidence that pacifier use reduces the risk of SIDS (sudden infant death syndrome). We recommend using a one-piece pacifier to decrease the risk of choking. If your baby is fussy, shows no clear signs of hunger, and giving a pacifier seems to be soothing, then great! If, however, your baby spits it right out and demonstrates hunger cues, your baby may be hungry. With all this said, some babies may just not "take" to a pacifier.

We do recommend weaning the use of the pacifier by around 6 months of age, as the longer you wait, the more difficult it will be. We have all seen 3-year-olds who have no fewer than three pacifiers attached to them at all times. Let's try to avoid this!

How do I prepare for returning to work?

If you intend to return to work before weaning your baby, it is helpful to plan ahead for how you will continue to provide breast milk for your baby. You don't want to be looking for a room to pump in on your first day of work only to discover that other employees have booked the space or there is no place to pump. If you are not self- employed, it is helpful to discuss the range of accommodations with your supervisor or colleagues before you return to work. Most offices do have places to pump and store your milk. If not, remember that you have a legal right to express milk at work. If your employer has more than fifty employees and no place to pump, offer to help them figure out how to comply with the amendment to the Fair Labor Standards Act (FLSA), which was put into place when the Patient Protection and Affordable Care Act (ACA) was signed, and requires an employer to allow breaks and provide a place (other than a bathroom) for a mother to pump until her child is one year old. If your employer has fewer than fifty employees and can't accommodate these rules due to undue hardship, they are not legally obligated to follow this regulation, but you might be able to help them figure out how to accommodate your need to pump.

A great source for more information is the Department of Labor's face sheet on break time for nursing mothers (www.dol.gov/whd/nursingmothers/faqBTNM.htm). Your state may also have laws for your protection.

A provision within the ACA requires most health insurances, with some exceptions, to cover the cost of breast pumps and lactation consultants, too. It is helpful to contact your insurance company in advance of your due date, even if you are unsure of whether you will use the pump right away, so you know how to access the coverage that you are entitled to within your plan. Insurance plans usually list which pumps are covered on their website. Since the quality and type of pumps that are covered varies considerably, we find

Checklist for Returning to Work

- Do you have a breast pump and are you comfortable using it?
- How can you arrange for flexibility in your schedule to pump during the day?
- Does your work have an on-site day care center?
  - If so, do you want to feed your baby there?
  - Or do you prefer to pump and bring milk to your baby?
- Is there a room where you can pump?
- Where can you store your expressed breast milk and pump parts?
- Where can you clean your pump parts?
- How will you store and transport breast milk?

it helpful to compare the pumps covered by your plan and also seek out the opinions of lactation consultants and your health care providers to determine which pump might be best for you. Once you have an idea which model you may want, check to determine whether the manufacturer will help you get the pump through your insurance company. Many do. In some circumstances you may need to rent a more efficient pump than you can buy. Some hospitals, baby stores, and breastfeeding specialty shops rent pumps, and again, may provide you with information to help you seek reimbursement from your insurance company. Once you have your pump, it is also important to test it out so you are comfortable using it before your first day of work. Finally, we suggest having bottles, storage bags, and a cooler on hand to transport your milk.

When and how do I introduce the bottle?

Once breastfeeding is well established, which can take anywhere from a few days to a few weeks depending on your child, we recommend giving a bottle once every couple of days, if a parent wants their baby to be comfortable with bottle feeding. We suggest introducing the bottle at a much earlier time before the mom is going to be out of the house for long periods because we have found that if the bottle is introduced for the first time right before mom goes back to work, some babies will refuse the bottle all together, making an already difficult transition for mothers even more stressful. Practice also gives other caregivers and the baby a chance to interact and bond with each other before a mother starts leaving for work on a regular basis.

It is best to tap the baby's lips with the bottle nipple to encourage the baby to open his/her mouth and accept the nipple. Gently guide the nipple into the baby's mouth. Never force feed it, so that frustration and any negative associations with a bottle are minimized. If your baby initially rejects the bottle, placing a few drops of milk on his/her lips can be helpful to prepare your child for feeding. Sometimes babies aren't as willing to accept a bottle if they see or smell their mother in the same room. It the baby refuses to take a bottle from mom or while mom is in the same room, then it might be easier if mom leaves while another caretaker gives the bottle. On the other hand, some babies will accept a bottle more easily if it is wrapped in a piece of clothing that the mom has already worn. If a baby is still refusing the bottle, sometimes offering a bottle about an hour after a feeding, when your baby is hungry but not too full, and is more relaxed, might ease the introduction. If the baby refuses the initial type of bottle, it is helpful to buy a few different bottles and nipples to determine which one the baby prefers (don't be surprised, though, if the baby goes back to the original bottle you had). It takes practice and may take several days, but your baby will often get the hang of the bottle with some patience. Please see the bottle section for specific recommendations on how to choose a bottle for your child.

What are the current thoughts on banked breast milk?

Well-intentioned mothers often offer extra expressed breast milk to other parents on parent blogs, on internet groups, or to friends in their community. Although we do recommend breast milk for infants, we do not recommend giving a baby breast milk that has not been thoroughly tested and safely handled. Breast milk could possibly transmit HIV (if the donor is HIV positive) and other infections, could lead to side effects from medicines or drugs the donor has ingested, or if not handled and stored properly, may contain bacteria that could make a baby sick. Recent studies have shown that human milk found on internet sites had higher rates of contamination with bacteria and viruses. In addition, some human milk was not pure and had cow's milk added to it and often arrived warm or completely unfrozen.

Parents who want to feed human donor breast milk should have a detailed discussion with their pediatrician about where it is safest to obtain the milk; currently, there are more than a dozen human milk banks throughout the country with some type of safety standards in place. For example, the Human Milk Banking Association of North America (HMBANA, www.hmbana.org) guidelines are used in California and Texas while New York has its own rules over the operation and distribution of donor milk within the state. Although the FDA formed a working group on banked human milk, consisting of a panel of experts to gain more information on current practice guidelines, it currently does not guide or quality control the safety standards in place in human milk banks.

In some states, including Texas, California and Kansas, insurance companies may cover the cost of human donor milk, especially if it is being used for premature or other high risk infants. A good source of additional information on this topic is HMBANA, which provides lists of member banks and describes the screening and storage processes of donated breast milk.

If I decide to wean my baby, how long will it take and how do I do it?

Although the AAP recommends exclusive breastfeeding for approximately six months, after which breastfeeding is continued, along with complementary foods, until the baby is one year old and as long as desired thereafter, many mothers find they want or need to wean their babies earlier. There is no one perfect time to wean since weaning is a very personal decision. The process of weaning can take as little as a couple of weeks when a mother needs to quickly transition her baby to drinking formula from a bottle or may take many months (and sometimes over a year) when a mother chooses to allow her baby to gradually transition. If you want to wean your baby quickly, you can start by offering one bottle a day instead of breastfeeding. You can then try offering two bottles a day instead of breastfeeding after a couple of days, if your breasts feel comfortable and your baby has adapted to the bottle. If that goes well, you can continue to swap a breastfeed for a bottle feeding every couple of days until your baby is drinking exclusively from the bottle. If your baby is old enough to drink from a cup, you can skip bottles entirely and wean to a cup directly. It is usually easiest to eliminate your baby's favorite feeding last, such as the feeding before bedtime. Do not pump during these bottle feedings, so that your milk production will decrease and soon stop. If you experience engorgement, you may want to alleviate some of the pain by placing cool compresses on your breasts or using pain relievers, such as acetaminophen. Please reach out to your obstetrician, midwife, or your child's pediatrician to review what would work best for you.

Likewise, if you have been offering expressed breast milk either exclusively or partially and want to quickly wean from pumping, you can decrease your pumping in the same way that mothers drop feedings from the breast. Remove a pumping every couple of days, as long as your breasts feel comfortable. Continue until you are no longer pumping at all.

Some mothers are susceptible to clogged ducts when they drop breastfeeds or pumps. They may not be able to drop a full breastfeed or pump without discomfort and may need to gradually reduce the amount of time on the breast at a feeding or amount that they express when they pump. Cold compresses are often soothing when breasts are overly full. There are many products on the market, but you can make your own from bags of frozen peas or by pouring water in a disposable diaper and freezing it. Mothers used to be told to pump a little bit to "take the edge off" if they were uncomfortable during the weaning process. If they frequently "take the edge off" it merely stimulates the supply more. New knowledge has shown that it is often more effective for mothers to really drain their breasts thoroughly to remove the clogs once or twice a day until their breasts adapt to the reduced frequency of pumping or feeding.

No matter what age you wean your baby or how long or short it takes to do so, weaning is often an emotional time for most mothers. It can be helpful to seek support from other moms who are going through or who have already gone through the same process. Your baby will continue to need you just as much when he/she was breastfeeding, but will simply be entering a different phase.

Formulas

Although we do routinely recommend that new parents exclusively breastfeed whenever possible, we also tell parents that babies will grow and develop well on formula, too. Commercial infant formulas have been developed based on extensive research and with a baby's optimal health and development in mind, and formulas replicate the nutrition elements of human breast milk as closely as is possible. So while you may often hear health professionals say, "Breast is best," we recognize that infant formula is also a very acceptable alternative and parents who need or want to give formula to their infants should feel comfortable about doing so. This section discusses different types of formula and topics such as how to mix and store formula and how to choose the right formula for your baby.

There are a variety of different companies and formulas on the market and new ones are being added on a regular basis. They come in powder, concentrated,

Whey vs. Casein Protein

Traditional cow's milk protein formula contains 80 percent casein and 20 percent whey protein. Human breast milk contains more whey (approximately 70 percent) and less casein protein (approximately 30 percent). Some formulas try to adjust this percentage to mimic breast milk and are marketed as being easier for babies to digest. Examples of these formulas include Enfamil Gentlease, which has 60 percent whey and 40 percent casein, and Gerber Good Start, which has 100 percent whey protein. Again, the majority of infants will do well on traditional cow's milk protein formula, but it is important to realize that there are many formulas on the market.

Probiotics and Prebiotics

Probiotics ("good" bacteria and yeast) are live microorganisms that support the body's intestinal flora. Although generally safe, there is not enough evidence for the AAP to recommend routine addition of probiotics to all infant formulas.

Prebiotics are nondigestible food and fiber compounds that stimulate the growth of "good" bacteria in the intestines.

and ready-to-feed forms. All infant formulas contain similar calories and nutrients but may contain different types of proteins, fats, and sugars, and some may have additional supplements, such as probiotics or omega-3 fatty acids.

Why can I give my baby a cow's milk–based formula but not whole cow's milk?

Your child is not able to fully digest whole cow's milk and proteins in whole cow's milk can also irritate the digestive tract. Cow's milk does not contain adequate amounts of iron, linoleic acid (essential fats!), vitamins C and E, and other nutrients, and it contains excessive amounts of sodium, potassium, and protein. Cow's milk–based formula, however, is fortified with minerals and vitamins as well as proteins and fats that mimic human milk and allow your child to adequately grow.

The same is true for milk alternatives including soy milk. Cow's milk and milk alternatives can be started after your child is 1 year old.

Can I use a store-brand formula?

The chart on page 23 lists the names of the most popular brands, but there are over fifty store brand versions available that all provide similar safety, quality, and nutritional content. The FDA and AAP have both set guidelines and recommendations for the nutritional standards of all infant formula, for both store and national brands.

For a variety of reasons, most infants are started on popular brand-name formulas or continue on the formula offered in the hospital where a baby is born, although studies have shown that switching to comparable nonbrand versions is well tolerated. In addition, store-brand versions cost as little as one-third as much as the national brand equivalents.

Examples of Common Formula Types and Uses

NAME	INGREDIENTS AND USES	EXAMPLES
Cow's Milk Protein (purified from whole milk)	These formulas contain cow's milk protein in its complete form. They are usually the first formulas that are tried. The majority of infants will grow well on this type of formula.	Earth's Best Organic Enfamil Newborn Similac Advance Similac Non-GMO
Partially Hydrolyzed Protein	These formulas contain proteins that are partially broken down but can still contain larger milk proteins. They are marketed as being easier to digest.	Enfamil Reguline Gerber Good Start Similac Sensitive
Extensively Hydrolyzed Protein	These formulas contain proteins that are all broken down into small protein pieces. They are typically fed to infants with cow's milk protein allergy or milk protein–induced proctocolitis. They are also lactose free.	Enfamil Nutramigen Gerber Extensive HA Similac Alimentum
Amino Acid (available in powdered form only)	These formulas contain proteins that are broken down into the smallest protein unit, known as amino acids. They can be offered to infants with cow's milk protein allergy or milk protein–induced proctocolitis. They are also lactose free.	Alfamino Elecare Neocate Puramino
Soy	These formulas contain soy protein, but unlike cow's milk protein formulas, they are lactose-free. They are useful for some rare metabolic disorders (such as galactosemia) and temporarily after a diarrheal illness, if recommended by a physician.	Enfamil Isomil Gerber Good Start Soy Similac Isomil
Low-lactose or lactose-free	These formulas are lactose-free or contain minimal lactose. Lactose intolerance in infants is rare. Some infants may have transient lactose intolerance following a diarrheal illness. However, most children will not need to switch formulas following a diarrheal illness.	Similac Sensitive (virtually lactose free) Enfamil Gentlease (low lactose)

There are many reasons why we choose one formula over another. Personal experience and recommendations from our child's pediatrician or friends and family play an important role. It is your choice what brand of formula you decide to feed your child, but you can do so with the knowledge that quality and content is similar among the different brands.

Which formula is best for my healthy full-term infant?

For healthy full-term infants, pediatricians will suggest starting with a cow's milk–based formula, such as Enfamil Complete, Similac Advance, or the store-brand equivalent. There are also organic versions of these formulas available as well, such as Earth's Best Organic.

Which formula is best for my baby with cow's milk protein allergy?

Extensively hydrolyzed protein and amino acid-based formulas are known as "predigested" formulas because the protein components are already broken down. Extensively hydrolyzed protein formulas contain small peptide proteins, and in amino acid-based formulas, proteins are broken down to the smallest protein building blocks, known as amino acids. Both of these formulas are options for babies who have cow's milk protein allergy or milk protein–induced proctocolitis (discussed in detail later in this chapter). They tend to not taste as good as the complete cow's milk–based formulas, but fortunately taste buds are not fully developed during infancy and babies notice more of a difference in taste than a "bad" or "good" one. They also will gradually adjust to the new formula. These formulas, especially the amino acid–based ones, are typically more expensive, but may be covered by your insurance plan with a prescription from your physician. You should discuss these formulas with your pediatrician before starting them.

If there is a strong family history of allergies, which formula should I use?

So far, no studies have shown conclusive evidence that using formula is better than breastfeeding to prevent a baby from developing allergic conditions. So breastfeeding is recommended even by allergy experts. However, when breastfeeding or providing expressed breast milk is not an option, allergists do have some recommendations regarding formula choices. Despite limited research in this area, we recommend that for "allergy at-risk" babies (meaning there is a parent or sibling with food allergies or other significant allergy issues), if breastfeeding is not possible, a partial or extensively hydrolyzed–protein formula be given to the baby for at least the first six months of life, rather than a regular cow's milk formula.

Should I switch formulas?

Most children will do well on a traditional cow's milk protein formula. There are many formulas on the market that have different or added components, such as a different ratio of the milk proteins, casein and whey, low lactose, or added prebiotics or probiotics. Most of the time, these changes are made to mimic components of breast milk or to potentially improve digestion in babies who have colic, constipation, or gastroesophageal reflux. All additives to infant formulas are regulated by the FDA, which requires proof of safety and efficacy for each additive. The benefits of changing formulas, however, vary from child to child, so be sure to check with your pediatrician before switching formulas. Though we do not feel that using these formulas is usually medically necessary, we have provided you with a list of medical conditions for which formulas are usually marketed:

Colic: Colic usually begins at 3 weeks and resolves by 3 to 4 months of life. The cause of colic is not known, although increased gas is sometimes felt to be a contributing factor. Certain formulas have less lactose or are lactose-free (Similac Sensitive, Enfamil Gentlease, and partial and extensively hydrolyzed–protein formulas) or contain partially broken down whey protein (Gerber Good Start), which are thought to be easier to digest and may decrease gas production. Some of these formulas may also contain prebiotics (the majority of Similac formulas), while others contain probiotics (Gerber Good Start Gentle for Supplementing and Gerber Good Start Soothe), which may decrease gas and symptoms of colic.

Constipation: Formulas that contain prebiotics may be helpful to keep your child's stools softer and more regular. There are a variety of formulas that contain prebiotics. Enfamil Reguline, which contains partially hydrolyzed proteins, and traditional cow's milk protein formulas, such as Enfamil Infant and Similac Advance, all have added prebiotics.

Gastroesophageal Reflux (GER): Gastroesophageal reflux is nearly universal in babies and young children. Infants may spit up during, at the end, or after a feeding (see page 43 for a more detailed explanation of GER). Most children who are spitting up but growing well will not require any treatment or change in formula. Of the major infant formula brands, there are currently two different products on the market, Enfamil AR and Similac for Spit-up, where rice has been added to the formula to help decrease spit-up. Enfamil AR remains thin so you can still use a normal nipple and the formula will thicken in your child's stomach when it is exposed to stomach acid. Since Enfamil AR requires stomach acid to activate the rice to thicken, it may not be effective if your child is on medications that decrease stomach acid such as Zantac (ranitidine) and Pepcid (famotidine), which are histamine-2-receptor antagonists, or Prevacid (lansoprazole) and Nexium (esomeprazole), which are proton pump inhibitors. Similac for Spit-up is a little thicker from the get-go and will require more thorough mixing (though it will still be grainy!) and may require a larger nipple size. We recommend increasing by one nipple size or using a crosscut or Y-cut nipple with Similac for Spit-up. Please speak to your pediatrician to discuss whether your child would benefit from these formulas.

Stomach bug: Following a stomach bug with diarrhea, your child may not be able to digest lactose as effectively. Lactose is the typical sugar found in most infant formulas and in breast milk. Often your child should remain on their regular milk, but if your child has significant diarrhea, or his/her stomach is becoming gassy, bloated, or upset with his/her regular formula, your baby *may* benefit from a lactose-free or low-lactose formula for a few weeks. An example of this type of formula is Similac Sensitive. The course of diarrhea may be variable, though you may switch back to your child's regular milk usually within two to three weeks or when the stool pattern normalizes.

Are formulas made outside of the United States safe to use?

Some parents prefer to use formulas made in Europe and Australia. There are many popular brands such as Holle from Switzerland. You should consult with your pediatrician to ensure that the formula is imported legally into the United States and meets FDA requirements. If so, the formula should be safe to use.

Should I use a recipe I found on the internet to make my child's formula from scratch?

We do not recommend this for several reasons. It is very easy, especially when you are sleep deprived, to incorrectly mix the ingredients making up the homemade formula, which may result in electrolyte imbalances and malnutrition in your newborn. Homemade formulas may not contain all the nutrients and vitamins a baby needs, may be harder to digest, are not regulated by the FDA, and, if handled improperly, can cause a baby to ingest harmful bacteria.

How many calories are in formula and breast milk?

Most formulas when mixed contain approximately twenty calories per ounce. However, since it is estimated that breast milk contains between eighteen to twenty calories per ounce, some formulas (like Similac Advance) have changed the concentration so that they contain nineteen calories per ounce when mixed. One calorie is not a major difference, but can be important if your child is not gaining weight appropriately.

How do I mix the formula?

Follow the manufacturer's instructions on the packaging for your specific formula. Formulas come in three different forms: powder, concentrated, and ready-to-feed.

In most cases, when using powdered formula, you would mix two ounces of water with one level scoop of powdered formula. There are, however, exceptions to this rule. Neocate and PurAmino, amino acid–based formulas, for example, have a one-to-one ratio and one ounce of water is mixed with one scoop of formula. Also, if your baby is a preemie, has certain chronic medical conditions, or is not gaining weight appropriately, your pediatrician may instruct you to mix the formula to increase the amount of calories in each ounce. If your baby needs to drink formula with increased calories, only do so under your pediatrician's direct guidance and instructions.

Concentrated formula should be mixed at a one-to-one ratio with water. Most containers come in thirteen-ounce bottles, so if you mix thirteen ounces of water with the entire contents, you will have twenty-six ounces of formula. This formula can be refrigerated for up to forty-eight hours. Alternatively, if you prefer to make one bottle at a time and want to make a 4-ounce bottle, you can add two ounces of the concentrate to two ounces of water and mix thoroughly.

Ready-to-feed formula is exactly what it sounds like. The formula should not be diluted with additional water and is ready to use!

It is important that you prepare formula exactly as directed. Making a more concentrated formula (by adding more powder than is recommended) or mixing a more diluted formula (by adding more water to than is recommended) can lead to serious health issues. Highly concentrated formula can lead to vomiting, constipation, excessive weight gain, and dehydration. The high protein content can also cause kidney problems. Diluted formula may lead to diarrhea, poor weight gain, and seizures due to low salt levels in the blood that can lead to brain swelling.

What type of water do I use to make powdered or concentrated formula?

It really depends on two factors: the quality of your tap water and whether your water is fluorinated.

If you live in an area with safe drinking water, you can prepare the formula with regular tap water without boiling it first. In this case, we don't recommend bottled water or "baby" water since it is expensive and unnecessary. If your water comes from a well, and may contain chemicals including nitrates, or if you are uncertain of the quality of your water, talk to your pediatrician about

How to Mix Formula

Powdered Formula

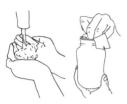

Thoroughly wash
hands, formula
container (if needed),
and all bottle parts.

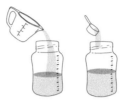

For every 2 ounces
of water, add 1 level
scoop of powder.
Water should be added
before powder.

Attach nipple
and cap and
shake to
combine.

Concentrated Formula

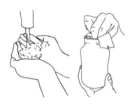

Thoroughly wash
hands, formula
container (if needed),
and all bottle parts.

Shake
formula well.

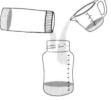

To make 2 ounces
of formula,
add 1 ounce of
concentrate to
1 ounce of water.

Attach nipple
and cap and
shake to
combine.

Ready-to-Feed Formula

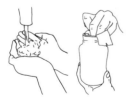

Thoroughly wash
hands, formula
container (if needed),
and all bottle parts.

Shake formula
well.

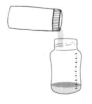

Pour desired
amount of formula
into bottle.

Attach nipple
and cap.

using bottled water or boiled tap water. If you use boiled tap water, boil for approximately one minute and let it cool before mixing it with the formula. If you are not sure about the quality of the tap water, you can contact your state's environmental agency or talk to your pediatrician about local guidelines.

It is also important to consider if the water you use is a source of fluoride. Since the 1940s, fluoride has been added to community tap water to help decrease the prevalence of tooth decay. Currently, two-thirds of the US population receives fluoride this way. If you are not sure, check with your local water board to see if your tap water is fluoridated. If not, your child may need supplementation after 6 months of life.

When preparing formula from powder or liquid concentrate, the American Dental Association states that you may use fluoridated tap water. Although fluoride is important in the development of strong teeth, excessive use of fluoridated water may contribute to the development of mild enamel fluorosis, a change in appearance of tooth enamel due to excessive fluoride exposure. Enamel fluorosis presents as faint white spots on teeth that are often difficult to even see. Fortunately, it does not interfere with the overall health of your child's teeth. If enamel fluorosis is a concern, review with your pediatrician the different sources of fluoride your child is receiving to discuss whether it may be useful to solely or occasionally use water low in fluoride to prepare the formula, which is labeled as deionized, purified, demineralized, or distilled.

How long does formula last?

A prepared bottle of formula can be kept at room temperature for no more than an hour. If the formula has been warmed, also keep it for no more than an hour, and do not rewarm it, as this increases the risk of harmful bacteria growth. By the same token, if the baby feeds from the bottle, but there is some milk left in the bottle, the leftover milk should be discarded after one hour and not be given again to the baby, since drinking from a bottle can actually introduce bacteria into the milk.

Once opened, unused ready-to-feed formula, concentrated formula, or formula made from concentrated formula, should be refrigerated and used within forty-eight hours. If you prepare the formula from powder, unused formula, once mixed, should be refrigerated and used within twenty-four hours.

Once a container of powdered formula is opened, it should be discarded after thirty days.

Recommended Duration of Use of Different Forms of Formula	
TYPE OF FORMULA	**DURATION OF USE**
Prepared bottle from any type of formula	Keep at room temperature for up to 1 hour. If bottle is warmed, discard in 1 hour and don't reheat it. If baby drinks from bottle, discard after 1 hour.
Opened, unused concentrated, or unused formula made from concentrated formula	Refrigerate and use within 48 hours.
Opened, unused ready-to-feed formula	Refrigerate and use within 48 hours.
Unused formula prepared from powder	Refrigerate and use within 24 hours.*
Opened container of powder formula	Discard after 30 days.

*There is a shorter duration of use with powdered infant formula since it's not sterile.

Can I switch among powder, ready-to-feed, and concentrated formulas?

Yes, you can switch between the different types of formula. They contain the same nutrients and calories and most children do well when switching between the different forms. Some children, however, may have difficulty tolerating the powdered version of the same formula that they are used to drinking in the ready-to-feed form. The reason for this intolerance is not well understood. However, some of the ready-to-feed forms, including Similac Alimentum, are corn-free while the powdered formulas may contain corn.

My child was born prematurely. Can I use regular formula and can I still breastfeed?

Premature infants can be fed breast milk, but may require additional calories, so milk fortification and special formulas are often necessary. Children born prematurely may also require different nutrients than children delivered at full term. They need higher amounts of calcium, phosphorus, protein, sodium, potassium, and other minerals including iron, zinc, and copper.

Fortification of breast milk with human milk fortifier, which increases the breast milk by two calories per ounce, is often necessary to provide the correct amount of nutrients, to allow a child to gain weight adequately.

There are also special formulas designed for premature babies. Infants may require these formulas during the first nine months of life, although this depends on a variety of factors such as birth weight and growth during the first year of life. Your baby's pediatrician will monitor your baby's growth closely to determine if and how long to stay on a special formula. Some examples of these formulas include Enfamil Enfacare and Similac Neosure.

Common Birth Definitions

- **Early Term:** A baby born between 37 and 39 weeks of pregnancy.
- **Full-term:** A baby born between 39 weeks and 41 weeks of pregnancy.
- **Later term:** A baby born between 41 and 42 weeks of pregnancy.
- **Post-term:** A baby born after 42 weeks of pregnancy.
- **Premature (preemie):** A baby born at less than 37 weeks of pregnancy.
- **Late pre-term:** A baby born between 34 and 37 weeks of pregnancy.
- **Moderately pre-term:** A baby born between 32 and 34 weeks of pregnancy.
- **Very pre-term:** A baby born between 28 and 32 weeks of pregnancy.
- **Extremely pre-term:** A baby born before 28 weeks of pregnancy.

Bottles and Nipples

Whether your baby is feeding with formula, expressed breast milk, or exclusively breastfeeding and using an occasional bottle, finding the right bottle for your baby can be quite challenging. There are dozens upon dozens on the market, and you'll have to use trial and error to find the one that works for your infant. This section gives an overview of bottles and also discusses the different types of nipples and when to switch among them.

Which types of bottles are available?

Going to a baby store and looking at a wall full of different types of bottles can be completely overwhelming! You might decide what you think is the best for your baby, but your little one might disagree. It is not uncommon to have to try out a few different brands before you find the perfect match for your baby and for you. Convenience and ease of use are also important considerations. For instance, some bottles have many parts and cleaning them several times a day for a year may be cumbersome. In general, smaller 2 to 4-ounce bottles are good first choices, and when the baby is taking more milk, at around 2 months, the bigger 8-ounce bottles will be needed. You should select a bottle that is practical for your baby, for your family, and for your lifestyle.

Here we have gathered some basic guidelines to help you choose:

Standard Bottles: These are the typical-shaped bottles with no bells and whistles, that are either completely straight or have minimally curved sides. These are the easiest to clean since they only include the bottle and the nipple and are often less costly.

Anti-gas Bottles: There are three popular options to reduce gas: disposable liners, natural flow system, and angle-neck bottles.

- **Disposable liners:** These bottles are marketed as more convenient with less cleanup time. They have presterilized disposable liners that collapse when the baby sucks to prevent air from mixing with the milk, and therefore, are supposed to reduce a baby's gassiness. Some examples are Playtex Premium nurser with drop-in liners and Philips nurser.
- **Natural flow system:** These contain a vent system inside the bottle that creates positive pressure flow and vacuum-free feeding to eliminate air bubbles in the milk and to mimic breastfeeding. This system is marketed to help colic, gas, and spit-up. Some examples are Dr. Brown's and Tommee Tippee.

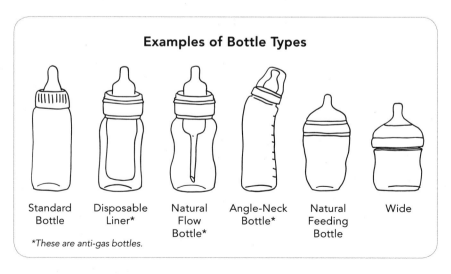

Examples of Bottle Types

| Standard Bottle | Disposable Liner* | Natural Flow Bottle* | Angle-Neck Bottle* | Natural Feeding Bottle | Wide |

*These are anti-gas bottles.

- **Angle-neck bottles:** These are bent at the neck, marketed to be easier for both baby and caregiver to hold and allow for the baby to be fed in an upright or semi-upright position. This design helps keep the nipple filled with liquid, not air, and is supposed to make the baby less gassy. Some examples are Evenflo Advanced Angled Bottle and Playtex BPA Free Ventaire Bottle.

Natural Feeding Bottles: These bottles are marketed to mimic the texture of mom's breast and nipple in the baby's mouth, and to make it easier for babies to transition from breast to bottle. Some examples are Tommee Tippee, Lansinoh mOmma Feeding Bottle, and Comotomo Natural Feel.

Wide Bottles: These bottles have both straight and angled shapes and have a wider neck and base on the nipple. The wider base of the nipple is marketed to more closely resemble mom's areola and nipple, and therefore, to help transition from a breast to a bottle. Some examples are Dr. Brown's wide-neck bottles and Born Free wide-neck glass bottle.

And what do we think? There is no perfect bottle or one "it" bottle that all pediatricians recommend. Personally, some of our children have done well with Dr. Brown's bottles while others have done well with Playtex. We usually recommend the bottles that have worked for us. It is all about trial and error and every baby is different; we suggest buying a few of the different types of bottles and seeing which one works best for you and your baby.

Do I have to sterilize bottles every time I use them?

The first time you use a bottle and nipple, they should be boiled for about five minutes or according to the manufacturer's instructions. After this initial use, you can clean all bottle parts thoroughly under hot soapy water and rinse the parts until they are free of soap. You can also clean them in the dishwasher with the hot water setting. Of course, there are also specialized bottle sterilizers, which are convenient but not needed.

What do the different levels of nipples mean and how do I know when to switch?

Most of the bottle manufacturers generally have the same type of levels for their nipples. Level one is for 0- to 3 month-olds and provides a slower milk flow, level two is for 3- to 6 month-old babies and provides a medium milk flow, level three is for 6-plus-month-olds who prefer a fast flow, and level four is for 9-plus-month-olds and has a fast flow (level four may not be needed if your

Definition of Different Nipple Levels

NIPPLE LEVEL	TYPE OF FLOW	RECOMMENDED AGE
Level one	Slow flow	0–3 months
Level two	Medium flow	3–6 months
Level three	Fast flow	6+ months
Level four	Faster flow	9+ months

baby has transitioned to a sippy cup). Many companies also sell nipples for premature babies and a Y-cut or crosscut nipple for thicker fluids, for example, if your baby has reflux and your pediatrician recommends thickening your baby's milk with cereal.

When do you switch between the levels? Just because your baby turned 3 months old, doesn't necessarily mean you need to switch right away to a level two nipple. If feeding is going well with the level nipple you are currently using, you can still continue with that nipple. If your baby is gagging on the milk, much of it is dripping out of his mouth, or the flow appears too fast, try switching to a lower level nipple. As your baby becomes older and is more adept at sucking, if he/she seems to be taking a while longer (more than twenty minutes) to finish the bottle or is becoming frustrated at the bottle, switching to a higher level may prove beneficial.

Real Life Parenting

When Anthony's son Sebastian was 2 months old, he was drinking two to three ounces of milk at a time and looked uncomfortable and arched his back at the middle and end of each feeding. Anthony thought these might be signs of gastroesophageal reflux, but noted that Sebastian was not spitting up and he seemed to still be hungry at the end of the feeding. Anthony decided to try to increase the nipple level. This change led to an increase in both comfort and volume during each feeding. If your baby seems uncomfortable during feeds, you may want to consider a change in nipple levels.

Expected Growth

All parents want to ensure that their newborns are growing at the proper rate. During these first few months, pediatricians see babies on a regular basis to keep close track of a baby's weight gain and development. This section discusses what the normal expected growth of a baby is and if parents need to buy a home scale to monitor their baby's weight gain.

What is the normal expected growth of a baby?

Since infants eat every few hours during the first few months of life, it is not surprising that this is also the stage when their weight increases at a faster rate. Your child will be weighed and measured at each well-baby visit. We included growth charts for your reference on page 220. Currently, it is recommended that the World Health Organization (WHO) growth charts be used until 2 years of life for all infants. The Centers for Disease Control and Prevention (CDC) growth charts are used after 2 years of age. The WHO growth chart was created in 2006 and is believed to better represent growth of the breastfed infant and normal physiological growth during infancy. You should ask your doctor which growth chart is being used, especially if you are breastfeeding and it appears that your child is not gaining weight appropriately. The WHO charts were created using data from a larger sample size of infants and better represents how infants should grow under ideal conditions. It includes infants from a variety of ethnicities.

An easy way to gauge if your child is gaining weight appropriately is to consider the *rule of one ounce*. Your baby should gain approximately:

- 1 ounce per day from birth to 3 months;
- 1 ounce every other day from 3 to 6 months;
- 1 ounce every three days from 6 to 12 months.

In addition, your child's length should increase by approximately $1/2$ to 1 inch per month and head circumference should increase by $3/4$ inch per month during infancy.

When Do Growth Spurts Occur?

You may notice your child is feeding more frequently during certain growth spurts, which usually occur when they are about 2 weeks, 3 weeks, 3 months, 6 months, and 9 months old.

What is a growth percentile?

At every well-baby visit, your doctor will plot your child's weight, height, and head circumference on a growth chart to determine your baby's percentile. A percentile gives an idea of where your child's growth compares to other children who are the same age and sex. For example, a boy with a weight at the 10th percentile indicates that the boy weighs more than 10 percent and weighs less than 90 percent of boys his age. Remember that the number itself is not as important as is consistent growth along a similar percentile over time.

What do I need to do to ensure that my child is growing well? Should I buy a scale?

In short, we do not recommend purchasing a scale. It may lead to unnecessary anxiety and stress. A baby's weight may fluctuate throughout the day; if the weight is taken right after a feeding, the baby may be a few ounces heavier than if it is taken later on in the day right after a bowel movement or before a feeding. Your home scale is also likely to vary from your pediatrician's scale, and you may worry when your baby's weight does not match what was measured in your pediatrician's office. It is best, therefore, to resist the temptation to monitor your baby's weight at home and to just have your baby weighed at his/her regular doctor appointments on one consistent scale. If your infant is eating, stooling, and urinating well, you should feel reassured he/she is likely getting enough nourishment to grow well. Your baby will see the pediatrician a few days after going home, then at 1 to 2 weeks old, and again at 1 month of age. Of course, if you are concerned about your baby's feeding and

Real Life Parenting

We know how hard it is not to look at a baby's daily weight as a victory or failure for us as parents. When Sebastian was born, Anthony had a scale and weighed him every day. He was happy when Sebastian gained an ounce or two and worried on days when Sebastian did not gain or lost weight from the previous day. He knew that Sebastian was happy, eating, stooling, and had normal wet diapers, but he became focused on the number on the scale. After the two-week visit, Anthony removed the scale from his home. The scale will never return when he has a second child because it caused unnecessary worry, even though he knew better.

growth, you can schedule an appointment to see your doctor earlier, but try to keep the equipment outside of your home.

Medical Concerns

There are a few common medical conditions related to nutrition that we often see arise during a baby's first few months. Even though your baby may not be experiencing one of these conditions now, or may never experience them, we find it is helpful to know what to expect and to be prepared in case these symptoms do occur. Of course, we always recommend talking to your pediatrician before following any course of action. Here we discuss the different forms of milk allergy, gastroesophageal reflux, and constipation. These common topics will be discussed in older age groups as well, since the treatment may be different depending on the age of your child, and are also discussed again in greater detail in chapter 6.

Milk Allergy or Intolerance

Some babies may have an intolerance or allergy to cow's milk protein. The most common milk intolerance seen in infants is cow's milk–induced proctocolitis. There are other less common forms of cow's milk allergy, such as immediate gastrointestinal hypersensitivity (IgE-mediated milk allergy), that can also present in young babies. Below are descriptions of cow's milk–induced proctocolitis, and immediate gastrointestinal hypersensitivity (IgE-mediated milk allergy).

What is cow's milk–induced proctocolitis?

Cow's milk–induced proctocolitis, or allergic proctocolitis, is commonly called "cow's milk protein allergy" but is really a gut intolerance to milk or soy protein and is different from other forms of milk allergy. It generally occurs in the first few months of life, and as early as 2 to 3 weeks of life. It can be seen in formula-fed infants, but more commonly occurs in breastfed infants who are reacting to proteins from the mom's diet that make it into her breast milk. The hallmark symptoms are loose, mucousy stools, and flecks or streaks of blood in the stool. Sometimes bowel movements are more frequent and your child may have increased gastroesophageal reflux symptoms, including spit-up. More often a baby with allergic proctocolitis is healthy, happy and otherwise thriving. This type of milk protein intolerance is not associated with severe vomiting, rashes, or hives. The diagnosis is primarily based on observed symptoms, but if present, your pediatrician may refer you to a gastroenterologist who may analyze your baby's stool for microscopic, or "occult," blood or for the presence of inflammatory allergy cells called eosinophils.

Treatment requires the removal of whole cow's milk protein. This may mean switching to an infant formula that contains broken-down milk proteins, such as an extensively-hydrolyzed protein or amino acid–based infant formula, which are also soy-free. Breastfeeding mothers will need to completely remove cow's milk and soy proteins from their diet (for infants who have this form of milk protein allergy, 30 to 50 percent will have the same reaction when exposed to soy).

Symptoms will generally improve three to five days after the formula is changed or after a mother eliminates milk and soy from her own diet. Mothers should also not give their babies stored breast milk that was pumped before the dietary restrictions were in place. The great news is that allergic proctocolitis is treatable and the majority (greater than 95 percent) of children will outgrow this type of allergy by 9 to 12 months of life, without any long-term effects. If symptoms do not resolve when milk and soy are restricted, or if they recur upon reintroduction of milk products between 9 months and 1 year of life, a referral to an allergist or gastroenterologist may be indicated. Some children do have a more persistent form of allergic proctocolitis and may need to continue to avoid milk and soy products until 18 to 24 months of age.

What foods do I need to eliminate from my diet if I am breastfeeding and my baby has allergic proctocolitis?

As previously stated, you will probably be instructed to avoid both cow's milk and soy. Following a milk-free diet means that you should remove all dairy products as well as products that contain milk protein. For a soy-free diet, you also need to avoid soy and soy protein. Conveniently, in the United States there is a law that requires food manufacturers to clearly label milk and soy in the ingredient list. Milk proteins can show up in surprising places, even in "nondairy" and lactose-free products. "Nondairy" may still contain milk-derived ingredients. For somebody with a severe milk allergy, this can be a problem, but someone with lactose intolerance should be able to tolerate it. "Dairy-free" is more likely to be safe, but it is not a regulated labeling term, and these products can contain milk. Reading ingredient labels is always essential! Milk may also be identified as a milk protein on a label (such as casein, lactalbumin, whey, or lactulose). Soy may initially seem easy to avoid, but soy is an ingredient in a lot of processed foods, and you will need to read ingredient labels carefully to totally avoid soy. Of note, *highly refined* soybean oil and soy lecithin generally do

Sources of Calcium Other than Dairy

- Dark green leafy vegetables (such as broccoli, kale, collard greens, arugula)
- Calcium-fortified foods (such as orange juice, cereal, bread)
- Nuts (such as almonds) and beans (such as white beans)
- Fish (such as sardines, salmon)

Treatment of Allergic Proctocolitis

APPROPRIATE TREATMENT OPTIONS	INAPPROPRIATE TREATMENT OPTIONS
Amino acid–based formula (Alfamino, Neocate, Elecare, Puramino)	Partially hydrolyzed formula (Gerber Good Start)
Extensively hydrolyzed formula (Alimentum, Nutramigen)	Soy-based formulas (Prosobee, Isomil)
Maternal elimination diet (if breastfeeding)	Milk substitutes (soy, coconut, or almond milk)

not contain enough soy protein to cause a reaction, and it is very likely that you will be able to keep these particular soy ingredients in your diet. While it may be overwhelming at first to avoid dairy and soy, remember that you can usually still maintain beef, poultry, seafood, fruits, vegetables, nuts, beans, and all grains in your diet. Also, remember that allergic proctocolitis will typically resolve, so this diet will only need to be followed temporarily.

It is important, however, for breastfeeding mothers to make sure that they are getting enough calcium in their diet, which can be a challenge when they are avoiding dairy (see "Sources of Calcium Other Than Dairy" on p. 39). The recommended daily intake of calcium for breastfeeding moms is 1000 milligrams per day. If you have any questions about this diet, do not hesitate to seek out the advice of a registered dietitian.

When can I start introducing food back into my diet and my child's diet if my child has allergic proctocolitis?

Approximately six months after a diagnosis of allergic proctocolitis, or when the baby is about 9 to 12 months old, milk, soy, or any other implicated food can be gradually tried at home. This means reintroducing it into the breastfeeding mother's diet or directly into the baby's diet. Since allergic proctocolitis involves a delayed reaction to a food protein, you will need to continue to give the milk (or soy) and observe the baby for a delayed reaction. If the stool symptoms, such

---

Most Common Milk Ingredients to Be Avoided in Children with Immediate Allergic Reactions to Cow's Milk

- Casein
- Curds
- Lactalbumin
- Lactoferrin
- Lactoglobulin
- Lactose
- Lactulose
- Milk powder
- Rennet
- Whey

Aslo see page 224 for tips on avoiding your allergen.

---

as blood in the stool, recur, your pediatrician will generally recommend that you again eliminate the milk and soy (it will take several days for the stool to return to normal), and will determine a later time to do this food "trial" again. If the child develops symptoms again at that time, we usually recommend continuing the milk- and soy-free diet until the child is 18 months old and trying reintroduction at that time. Again, always speak with your pediatrician before having your baby try a food that you have been previously told to avoid.

It is also important that you introduce other complementary solid foods into your baby's diet. You do not need to wait until allergic proctocolitis resolves before giving your baby other new and age-appropriate foods. Allergic proctocolitis is *not* an indication for you to delay the introduction of solid foods beyond 6 months of age.

What is an immediate gastrointestinal hypersensitivity milk allergy?

Immediate gastrointestinal hypersensitivity (IgE-mediated milk allergy) is a type of milk allergy with symptoms occurring immediately or within minutes after exposure to milk, although symptoms can in some rare cases be delayed several hours. Symptoms may just include vomiting, but can also include rashes such as hives and respiratory symptoms such as coughing, wheezing, and sleepiness. This type of allergy to milk can be very severe, and may be present in a child who has other food allergies (such as eggs, soy, wheat, peanuts, tree nuts, fish, and shellfish). For infants with this type of milk allergy, close follow-up by an allergist is suggested, and reintroduction of milk at home is *never* recommended. Please see page 204 for more details on the symptoms and treatment of IgE-mediated allergies.

Infants who have a true IgE-mediated cow's milk allergy should not be exposed to other mammalian milks such as goat's milk or sheep's milk, as these animal milks may not be nutritionally sound for this age, are highly cross-reactive with cow's milk, and can cause an allergic reaction.

For an infant with immediate allergic reactions to cow's milk, it is important to avoid feeding the infant not only milk, but also all products that contain milk as an ingredient. All FDA-regulated manufactured food products that contain milk as an ingredient are required by law to list *milk* on the product label, so it is important to read all product labels carefully before feeding something new to your baby (please see chart on page 40).

Common Allergy Terms

Eczema is inflamed skin (or dermatitis) and may appear as dry, red, itchy patches, and fluid-filled blisters (vesicles), which can crust over. Eczema can range from very mild, with only a few patches of skin involved, to severe eczema that covers most of the skin's surface. *Atopic dermatitis* is the medical term for eczema that has an allergic trigger (for example, food or environmental allergens). Eczema is usually a chronic skin problem with periods of "flare-ups." Childhood eczema generally does improve or even resolve as children get older.

Hives (or urticaria) are raised pale or pink wheals (or welts) surrounded by a flat pink area of skin. People can develop a single hive or may develop hives all over their body. In some cases, hives may coalesce so that it is hard to identify an individual welt. Hives are caused by *histamine*, a natural chemical that is released by some skin cells. It is also responsible for itchiness. (This is why "antihistamines" are used to treat hives and other itchy allergic symptoms.) Hives can be a symptom of an allergic reaction, but can often develop with viral illnesses, including the common cold. Hives can be extremely itchy and uncomfortable, but hives themselves are not dangerous. Diphenhydramine (Benadryl), which is an antihistamine, can help relieve hives (see page 209 for dosing). Your doctor may also prescribe other antihistamines, such as cetirizine or loratadine. Hives may, however, present along with other symptoms of a more serious allergic reaction known as anaphylaxis.

Anaphylaxis is a serious allergic reaction that involves more than one system of the body. Symptoms usually start within five to thirty minutes after being exposed to an allergen (such as a medication, food, insect sting, or latex) but can take as long as several hours to develop. Some signs of anaphylaxis may include hives all over the body, swelling of the throat and trouble swallowing, swelling of other body parts, coughing, wheezing, chest tightness and pain, difficulty breathing, vomiting, diarrhea, pale skin, and fainting. Anaphylaxis is a medical emergency and can be fatal if not treated promptly with epinephrine (see page 210). Anyone who has an anaphylactic reaction should be taken to a hospital immediately for observation and treatment.

IgE (Immunoglobulin E) is a type of immunoglobulin (or antibody) that circulates in the blood or is attached to special cells in the skin, respiratory tract, or gut. IgE plays a role in many allergic conditions, including asthma, hay fever, and food allergies. People with allergic conditions often have higher than normal levels of total IgE circulating in the blood. Allergy testing often involves measuring specific IgE levels in the blood for things like foods, pollen, animals, dust mites, insect venom, or latex.

Spit-Up and Gastroesophageal Reflux

Babies can spit up a whole lot in the beginning! Most of the time the biggest issue is all the laundry that needs to be done, but it is still not fun to see your little one spit up what appears to be all he/she just ate. It is not always easy for parents to tell when spit-up is normal and when it is more severe and considered gastroesophageal reflux disease. This section discusses gastroesophageal reflux and gastroesophageal reflux disease, including causes, symptoms, and treatment options.

What is gastroesophageal reflux (GER)? What is the difference between GER and gastroesophageal reflux disease (GERD)?

Acid is normally produced in the stomach to aid in the digestion of food. Unlike GERD (gastroesophageal reflux disease) commonly seen in adults, GER (gastroesophageal reflux) in infants does not include a "D" because it is considered normal or physiologic, and not a disease. An ineffective lower esophageal sphincter (LES), the muscle located at the bottom part of the esophagus, is what causes gastroesophageal reflux. This muscle can open at random times in infants (known as transient relaxations), so if there is food in the stomach, spitting

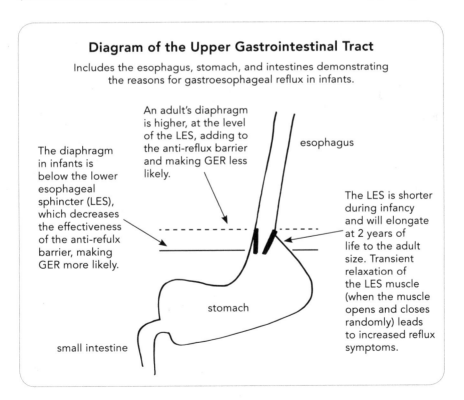

Diagram of the Upper Gastrointestinal Tract

Includes the esophagus, stomach, and intestines demonstrating the reasons for gastroesophageal reflux in infants.

An adult's diaphragm is higher, at the level of the LES, adding to the anti-reflux barrier and making GER less likely.

esophagus

The diaphragm in infants is below the lower esophageal sphincter (LES), which decreases the effectiveness of the anti-refulx barrier, making GER more likely.

The LES is shorter during infancy and will elongate at 2 years of life to the adult size. Transient relaxation of the LES muscle (when the muscle opens and closes randomly) leads to increased reflux symptoms.

stomach

small intestine

up and vomiting can occur. The muscle is also smaller and does not fully grow to the size as seen in adults until two years old. In addition, the diaphragm in infants is lower than in adults, making the anti-reflux barrier less effective.

GER usually starts at approximately 2 to 3 weeks of life and peaks between 4 to 5 months. The majority of infants will have complete resolution of symptoms by the time they are 9 to 12 months old. Children who have GER are usually known as "happy spitters." Happy spitters are not in pain when they spit up; they typically eat well and gain weight well. Some children with GER, however, may have increased congestion after feeding. Use of normal saline drops for babies may be useful if the congestion affects a child's sleep or if his/her milk intake decreases.

The "D" in GERD is added when there are complications, such as feeding problems, weight loss, and pain from esophagitis (irritation in the esophagus from acid), or lung issues that can occur if the reflux causes irritation in the lungs when some of the stomach contents are aspirated (this is very rare).

What are symptoms of GERD?

Symptoms of GERD include poor weight gain, frequent regurgitation, feeding refusal, crying with feeding, arching of the back, and vomiting and may be difficult to distinguish from physiologic reflux (GER, without the D). These symptoms may require further workup, including blood work and imaging studies, such as an upper gastrointestinal series (an X-ray to look at the anatomy of the esophagus, stomach, and intestines).

What is the treatment of GERD?

Treatment options at this age include frequent burping and keeping your child upright for up to thirty minutes after feeding. Some children may benefit from thickening formula or expressed breast milk by adding infant cereal (rice or oatmeal) to the bottle, which may decrease spit-up symptoms. Use of medications is indicated in children with weight loss, feeding problems, and esophagitis (inflammation in the esophagus) as a result of acid irritation. There are a variety of medical therapies available, including medicines that neutralize acid, decrease acid production, and block the release of acid. Discuss the risks and benefits with your physician before starting any long-term therapy for reflux, changing formulas, or changing mom's diet if breastfeeding. Please see page 194 for an expanded explanation of gastroesophageal reflux.

Spit-Up Versus Vomit

Spit-up occurs when breast milk or formula from the stomach reenters the esophagus and dribbles out of a baby's mouth or nose.

Vomiting is a more forceful emptying of the stomach contents through the mouth.

Constipation

Before a baby is born, most adults rarely talk about poop. A few minutes after a baby is born, it becomes all about the poop! One of the most common calls to a pediatrician or pediatric gastroenterologist is over concerns that a baby might be in pain when having a bowel movement or is having infrequent or hard stools. This section discusses what constipation is and what the normal stool patterns and colors of bowel movements should be at this age.

My baby looks like he is in a lot of pain when he is having a bowel movement. Is he constipated?

Constipation is a common problem in children and is defined as a change in normal bowel movements, including less frequent stools, larger stools, and increased pain with the passage of hard stool. It can also be associated with occasional streaks of blood on the outside of the stool and a change in appetite. At birth, and usually within the first 48 hours of life, infants will pass meconium. Delay of meconium passage (after 48 hours) warrants an evaluation by your pediatrician who may recommend a referral to a specialist.

Infants will usually stool with every feeding primarily due to the rapid movement of food through the colon and a strong gastrocolic reflux (which promotes stooling every time food enters the stomach). Stooling is considered involuntary since babies do not have control of the external anal muscle and the internal anal muscle opens automatically when stool causes the colon to stretch. In infancy, rectal confusion can occur. When infants push to pass a stool when they are lying down, the pelvic floor muscles do not relax and the anorectal canal does not straighten, making stools more difficult to pass (think about how hard it would be to have a bowel movement while lying down!). Although an infant may appear uncomfortable (making a face, bringing legs to the chest, or turning red in the face), as if in pain, he will pass a soft stool. Rectal confusion is completely normal and usually resolves by 2 to 4 months of life.

Some babies, however, can often go *one week* without a bowel movement. This is normal and not a reason for concern, as long as the stool is soft, they are passing gas, not vomiting, and their belly is soft and not distended. Abdominal massage or bicycle leg exercises (moving your baby's knees to his/her chest in a bicycle-like motion) may be helpful in these infants, but we do not recommend rectal stimulation (placing a thermometer or cotton swab in the anus) or suppositories, unless discussed with your pediatrician. Occasionally, small amounts of prune juice may be given to help the baby pass a stool (discuss with your pediatrician the right amount for your baby). However, you should never dilute your child's formula with water as this may lead to electrolyte imbalances and cause vomiting and irritability.

What is normal stool consistency? What is normal stool color?

Stools may be soft, mushy, and yellow, brown, or green in color. The color and consistency of stool will vary in the first few months of life. Beginning at birth and for the first few days of life, your child will pass meconium, a black, tarlike, and sticky stool. After the meconium is passed, stools will change to a light brown or greenish color and will become less sticky. Green stool is often normal since the color is derived from bile, which is the fluid in the intestines that aids in digestion of fats. Typically in adults, the bile is converted by bacteria in the colon to a brown color. Since infants have a quicker transit time (food moves through the intestines and colon at a faster pace) and have less bacteria to convert bile to brown, the stool can be green in color. If you are breastfeeding, stools may appear to be the consistency of diarrhea, but these liquidlike stools are normal and may also look like creamy peanut butter with seeds. The stools of infants who are formula-fed will have a similar color but will be more formed. In addition, if you are breastfeeding and decide to transition to formula, your baby's stool will also become more formed and you may notice a change in frequency.

Colors that may warrant a discussion with your physician are red (may indicate blood from an allergy, blood from rectal fissures caused by passing hard stool, or blood from other causes), black stool (which may suggest digested blood), and gray or tan (which may indicate liver issues). If your infant is on an iron supplement, it is normal for his/her stools to be black-grayish in color.

Real Life Parenting

Dina will never forget the night she heard her husband, Derek, yell out for help while he was changing their daughter's diaper. As he was changing the baby girl's diaper, she again pooped and stool shot across the changing table, onto his shirt, and somehow not only landed on their dog's back but also up the baby's back, too. Derek was convinced that she was having diarrhea, but it was just part of being a normal newborn. On that day, the term "UTB" or up-the-backers was born in Dina's household.

Healthy Recipes for Parents

Many, but not all nursing moms, will find that breastfeeding will help shed those extra pounds gained during pregnancy—no gym membership required! Normally, breastfeeding moms are told to eat an extra 400 to 500 calories a day, but this can vary with activity levels and their medical history (see an example of a daily meal plan for breastfeeding moms on page 50). There is no special diet that needs to be followed; it is best just to eat a variety of healthy options full of protein, whole grains, dairy, fruit, and veggies to ensure that you are getting enough essential nutrients and vitamins such as calcium, vitamin D, iron, omega-3 fatty acids, and folic acid. Eating based on your culture is also important so your baby can "taste" the different flavors through your breast milk that they will later be exposed to when they start eating solid foods.

Although the nutrition in these recipes is based on lactating moms, the recipes can be eaten by parents (even if you are not breastfeeding) as well as older children. When we were up most of the night feeding a newborn, we wanted healthy, hearty meals that would take just minutes to make, with common ingredients that we didn't have to go far to find. We also highlighted the nutrients each recipe contains. Please see page 216 for a table summarizing important nutrients and their food sources.

For these recipes, we make the claim that a recipe is a "good source" of a certain nutrient when the serving size we list meets 10 to 19 percent of the Dietary Reference Intake (DRI) for lactating moms. We claim a recipe is an "excellent source" of a nutrient when the serving size listed meets 20 percent or more of the DRI for the lactating moms.

Real Life Parenting

After Dina delivered her first daughter, who weighed in at almost ten pounds, she assumed she would immediately lose the ten pounds that Julia weighed, and the rest of the forty pounds she gained would melt away with breastfeeding. Some mothers may have this experience, but Dina definitely did not. Although some of the initial weight came off quickly with breastfeeding, she had to maintain a healthy diet, along with regular exercise, to slowly lose the rest of the weight she had gained. Dina still hasn't quite lost all of the weight, but she definitely no longer feels guilty about it, since she is truly happy with all that she has accomplished—delivering and raising two daughters!

Eating Fish and Shellfish While Pregnant or Breastfeeding

Fish is an important part of a healthy diet. It is rich in protein and omega-3 fats, which help in the growth and development of a baby. The USDA recommends that pregnant and breastfeeding mothers consume eight and up to twelve ounces (two to three servings) of cooked fish each week. But remember, it is best to eat fish that are low in mercury such as salmon, shrimp, flounder, tilapia, trout, pollock, light canned tuna, cod, and catfish, since mercury can be harmful to the developing nervous system of a young baby. The fish that are higher in mercury and should be avoided are shark, swordfish, king mackerel, and tilefish. White (albacore) tuna should also be limited in a breastfeeding mom's diet to 6 ounces a week.

Red and Processed Meat

In 2015, a group from the World Health Organization (WHO) met to discuss the carcinogenicity of eating red unprocessed meat (for example, beef, veal, pork, lamb, or goat) and processed meat (meat that has been salted, cured, smoked or processed in other ways to increase its preservation and flavor). Meat processing may produce known or potential carcinogens, while cooking methods such as pan frying, grilling, and barbecuing may cause higher levels of these chemicals, too. The group found *associations* of colorectal and other cancers with high consumption of red meat (100 grams daily) or processed meat (50 grams daily). However, there is no evidence that eating red meat causes colorectal cancer. The group determined red meat as "probably carcinogenic" and processed meat as "carcinogenic" to humans. The report alarmed many meat lovers, but really needs to be taken into perspective! Meats are a good source of iron and nutrients, and these studies are still new and ongoing. We recommend eating a varied diet full of fruits and vegetables and not consuming red or processed meat on a daily basis. Until more conclusive research is done and official recommendations are made, meat on occasion is acceptable (so you can still enjoy your Sunday bacon once in awhile!).

Daily Meal Plan for Breastfeeding Moms

FOOD GROUP	BREASTFEEDING ONLY	BREASTFEEDING PLUS FORMULA	WHAT COUNTS AS A SERVING?
Dairy	3 servings	3 servings	1 cup milk, fortified milk substitute, or yogurt 1½ ounces natural cheese ⅓ cup shredded cheese 2 cups cottage cheese ½ cup ricotta cheese
Fats/Oils	6 servings	6 servings	1 teaspoon vegetable oil 1½ teaspoons mayonnaise 2 teaspoons tub margarine
Fruits	2 servings	2 servings	1 cup fruit or 100% fruit juice ½ cup dried fruit
Grains and Starches	8 servings	6 servings	1 slice bread 1 cup ready-to-eat cereal ½ cup cooked pasta, rice, oatmeal, or cereal 5 whole-grain crackers 5 cups popcorn 1 pancake 1 tortilla
Proteins	6 servings	5 servings	1 ounce lean meat, poultry, or seafood ¼ cup cooked beans or tofu ½ ounce nuts or seeds 1 egg 1 tablespoon nut butter 2 tablespoons hummus
Vegetables	3 servings	2 servings	1 cup raw or cooked vegetables 2 cups raw leafy vegetables (such as spinach or lettuce) 1 cup 100% vegetable juice

Adapted from the USDA

Pistachio-Toasted Salmon

This is a quick and healthy meal that fits perfectly into a busy parent's lifestyle. Throw this salmon together in fifteen minutes with a salad and a healthy carb, and you have a balanced and delicious lunch or dinner. A great tip is to pick up some sides of salmon next time you are at the supermarket to freeze for later. Begin defrosting in the refrigerator the night before you plan on making the fish. | MAKES 3 SERVINGS

Preheat the oven to 400°F.

Mix together the pistachios and dried cilantro. On a parchment paper–lined baking sheet, squeeze the lemons over the fish, then drizzle with the olive oil. Season the salmon with salt and pepper to taste. Press the pistachio mixture on top of the fish with your hands. Place in the oven for 15 to 20 minutes. Keep an eye on the salmon to make sure the pistachios do not burn (if they begin to burn, cover the salmon loosely with foil for the remainder of the cooking time). The salmon is done when it is opaque in the center and flakes when prodded with a fork.

Serve warm or store in the refrigerator for up to 3 days.

½ cup coarsely ground salted pistachios

1 teaspoon dried cilantro (may substitute parsley)

2 lemons

12 ounce salmon fillet

2 tablespoons extra-virgin olive oil

Salt and pepper

Prep time: 10 minutes

Cook time: 15 to 20 minutes

Excellent source for lactating moms of protein, vitamins B_{12} and E, and omega-3 fatty acids.

Good source for lactating moms of vitamin C, iron, and potassium.

NUTRIENTS PER SERVING FOR ADULTS/TODDLERS: 1 serving: 4 ounces fish/1 ounce fish • Calories 443.1/110.8 • Total Fat 33.8 g/8.5 g • Saturated Fat: 5.9 g/1.5 g • Protein: 27.6 g/6.9 g • Carbohydrates: 8.2 g/2.1 g • Fiber: 2.2 g/0.5 g • Sugar: 2.4 g/0.6 g • Vitamin B_{12}: 3.7 mcg/0.9 mcg • Vitamin C: 18.6 mg/4.6 mg • Vitamin E: 5.7 mg/ 1.4 mg • Calcium: 36.6 mg/ 9.1 mg • Folate: 46.9 mcg/11.7 mcg • Iron: 1.3 g/0.3 g • Sodium: 155.4 mg/38.9 mg • Omega-3 fatty acid: 3.1 g/0.8 g • Potassium: 660 mg/165 mg • Zinc: 0.9 mg/0.2 mg • **Provides 1 protein serving for children 1 to 3 years.**

Veggie and Cheese Mini Frittatas

These frittatas are a good source of protein and a perfect way to get your veggies and a healthy dose of vitamins and minerals in the morning. Coupled with a healthy carb, they make a great nutritious breakfast. We love them since they are so easy to eat on the go and the bite-size portions make them perfect for both you and your toddler. | MAKES 30 MINI FRITTATAS

½ red bell pepper, diced with seeds removed

1 cup spinach, finely chopped

½ small red onion, finely chopped

1 cup whole milk (can substitute with nonfat or unsweetened/unflavored soy or almond milk)

¾ cup feta cheese (can substitute with reduced fat)

5 large eggs, whisked

Prep time: 15 minutes

Cook time: 30 minutes

Excellent source for lactating moms of vitamins B₁₂, C, and K.

Good source for lactating moms of protein, vitamin A, calcium, iron, and zinc.

Preheat the oven to 350°F. Spray a mini muffin pan with cooking spray.

In a medium bowl, combine the bell pepper, spinach, and onion. In another bowl, whisk the milk, cheese, and eggs until thoroughly combined. Add the egg mixture to the vegetable mixture. Scoop 1 tablespoon of the mixture into each well of the mini muffin pan. Bake for about 30 minutes or until the top of each mini frittata is brown and the eggs are firm.

Wrap cooled frittatas individually in plastic wrap and refrigerate for up to 3 days or freeze for up to 1 month.

Note

We love the combo of spinach and bell peppers, but feel free to add 1½ cups of your favorite vegetables (mushrooms, tomatoes, asparagus, arugula, broccoli, kale, and sun dried tomato to name a few).

To make a larger frittata, spray an 8- or 9-inch springform pan or pie dish with cooking spray. Prepare the ingredients the same way and pour them into the springform pan. Bake for 45 to 60 minutes, or until the top is bubbly, light golden brown, and the middle does not jiggle. Cool for 10 minutes and serve warm.

NUTRIENTS PER SERVING FOR ADULTS/TODDLER: 1 serving: 5 mini frittatas with full-fat dairy options/3 mini frittatas with full-fat dairy options • Calories: 145.2/87.1 • Total Fat: 9.4 g/5.6 g • Saturated Fat: 4.9 g/2.9 g • Protein: 9.6 g/ 5.8 g • Carbohydrates: 5.4 g/3.2 g • Fiber: 0.7 g/ 0.4 g • Sugar: 4.1 g/2.5 g • Vitamin A: 155.7 mcg/93.5 mcg • Vitamin B₁₂: 0.9 mcg/ 0.5 mcg • Vitamin C: 25.7 mg/15.4 mg • Vitamin D: 57.9 IU/34.7 IU • Vitamin K: 19.7 mcg/ 11.8 mcg • Calcium: 169.4 mg/101.7 mg • Iron: 1.1. mg/0.6 mg • Sodium: 290.1 mg/174.1 mg • Zinc: 1.3 mg/0.8 mg • Provides ½ protein serving, ⅓ dairy serving, and ¼ vegetable serving for children 1 to 3 years.

Hearty Bean and Kale Soup

There is nothing more comforting after a long day than sitting down to a warm bowl of hearty soup. You will be amazed at how flavorful and delicious something so nutritious can be! | MAKES ABOUT 12 CUPS

Cook the sausage in a large Dutch oven or soup pot over medium-high heat for 5 minutes or until the sausage is completely cooked and no pink remains. Using a slotted spoon, remove the sausage from the heat and set aside on a plate. Do not clean out the Dutch oven. Reduce the heat to medium and add the onions to the fat left in the pot. Sauté the onions for 5 minutes or until they start to turn golden and translucent. Add the garlic and stir for 30 seconds. Pour in the broth and scrape the bottom of the pan to loosen all the remaining brown bits. After 1 minute, add the beans, cooked sausage, and kale. Bring to a boil and then reduce the heat to a simmer and cover. Simmer for 30 to 40 minutes or until the kale is tender.

Serve immediately or cool and refrigerate for up to 3 days or freeze for up to 2 months.

Note

We like using the food processor to finely chop the onions, since it saves time. We also find that if toddlers are eating the soup, they often don't like eating big pieces of onion and will try to pick it out.

1 pound beef or pork sausage (may substitute ham), cut crosswise in ½-inch-thick pieces or cubes

1 medium onion, finely chopped (see Note)

3 cloves garlic, minced

8 cups low-sodium chicken broth

1 (15 ounce) can cannellini beans, drained and rinsed

1 bunch kale, stems removed, roughly chopped (approximately 4 cups)

Prep time: 15 minutes

Cook time: 40 to 50 minutes

Excellent source for lactating moms of vitamins C and K.

Good source for lactating moms of protein, fiber, omega-3 fatty acid, and iron.

NUTRIENTS PER SERVING WITH SAUSAGE FOR ADULTS/TODDLERS: 1 serving: 1 cup/½ cup • Calories: 208.1/104.1 • Total Fat: 13.9 g/7 g • Saturated Fat: 4.9 g/2.5 g • Protein: 9.8 g/4.9 g • Carbohydrates: 10.5 g/5.2 g • Fiber: 3.3 g/1.7 g • Sugar: 0.7 g/0.3 g • Vitamin C: 27.7 mg/13.9 mg • Vitamin K: 158.1 mcg/79 mcg • Calcium: 68 mg/34 mg • Iron: 1.5 mg/0.8 mg • Omega-3 fatty acid: 0.16 g/0.08 g • Sodium: 461.3 mg/230.6 mg • **Provides ½ protein serving and ¼ vegetable serving for children 1 to 3 years.**

Easy Cheesy Burgers

Hamburgers are one of the quickest meals for busy parents who have little spare time to make a home-cooked meal. Lean meats used here provide an excellent source of iron while spinach packs a nutritional boost. Top off your burger with one of our favorite foods, avocado, to add in good fats, potassium, and fiber. | MAKES 6 (5-OUNCE) BURGERS OR 10 (2.5 OUNCE) SLIDERS

1 teaspoon olive oil

2 cups lightly packed spinach leaves, chopped

1½ pounds 90% lean ground beef (may substitute ground chicken)

1 egg, beaten

½ cup Italian-style bread crumbs

½ cup cheddar cheese

Salt and pepper (for older toddlers and adults)

6 whole-wheat hamburger buns

optional toppings: avocado, tomato, lettuce, and sauteed onions

Preheat the oven to 400°F

Heat the olive oil in a nonstick skillet over medium-high heat. Add the spinach and cook until wilted, about 2 minutes. Remove the spinach from the heat and let it cool.

In a large bowl, mix the ground meat, spinach, egg, bread crumbs, and cheese. Grate half an onion over the mixture, if desired. Mix until evenly combined.

Form the meat mixture into 6 patties (or 12 patties if making sliders) and season both sides of each patty with salt and pepper. Place on a parchment-lined cookie sheet and bake for 20 minutes or until the patties reach desired level of doneness. Place the burgers on a warm bun with optional toppings.

Refrigerate the cooked and cooled hamburgers for up to 3 days or freeze raw patties (can stack with parchment paper in between) for up to 3 months.

Prep time: 10 minutes

Cook time: 20 minutes

With no added options, excellent source for lactating moms of protein, vitamins B_{12} and K, iron, and zinc.

With no added options, good source for lactating moms of fiber, calcium, and omega-3 fatty acids.

Note

As a butcher in New York, Dina's father, Joseph DiMaggio, recommends using half ground steak and half chuck for a tastier burger.

NUTRIENTS PER SERVING FOR ADULTS/TODDLERS: 1 serving: 1 beef burger with bun and no optional items/2.5 ounce beef slider with 1/2 bun and no optional items • Calories: 374.1/187 • Total Fat: 16.5 g/8.3 g • Saturated Fat: 6.5 g/3.3 g • Protein: 29.4 g/14.7 g • Carbohydrates: 27.5 g/13.8 g • Fiber: 4.1 g/2.1 g • Sugar: 3.9 g/2 g • Vitamin B_{12}: 2.2 mcg/1.1 mcg • Vitamin K: 50.3 mcg/25.2 mcg • Calcium: 138.7 mg/69.3 mg • Iron: 4.0 mg/2.0 mg • Omega 3 fatty acids: 0.2 g/0.1 g • Sodium: 403.4 mg/201.7 mg • Zinc: 6.5 mg/3.3 mg • **Provides 1 carbohydrate serving, 2 protein servings, and ⅛ vegetable serving for children 1 to 3 years.**

Oatmeal Power Cookies

The minute our alarm, which for most of us is our babies, goes off in the morning, we are busy running around and rarely have time to think about ourselves. These oatmeal cookies, with a glass of milk or cup of yogurt, are an easy way to get in breakfast and are perfect for on-the-go parents. We love them simply because they are tasty and make no claims they will increase your milk supply. These cookies are also a good way to get picky eaters to enjoy breakfast—we have never seen a toddler turn down a cookie! | MAKES APPROXIMATELY 30 COOKIES

Preheat the oven to 350°F.

In a large bowl, mix together the oats, flour, cinnamon, baking powder, and salt. Mix the bananas, butter, peanut butter, raisins, and vanilla in a medium bowl. Pour the banana mixture into the flour mixture and mix until just combined, then mix in the chocolate chips. Let the mixture rest for 10 minutes.

Using a tablespoon, scoop the batter onto a parchment-lined baking sheet, leaving 1 inch between cookies. Bake for 20 minutes. Cool and serve or refrigerate for up to 2 days or freeze for up to 1 month.

1 cup old-fashioned oats

1 cup whole-wheat flour

½ teaspoon ground cinnamon

½ teaspoon baking powder

¼ teaspoon table salt

4 ripe bananas, mashed

¼ cup unsalted butter, melted

½ cup peanut butter (may substitute sunflower butter)

½ cup raisins

1 teaspoon vanilla extract

½ cup semi-sweet chocolate chips

Prep time: 15 minutes

Cook time: 20 minutes

Good source for lactating moms of fiber and iron.

NUTRIENTS PER SERVING FOR ADULTS/TODDLERS: 1 serving: 2 cookies/1 cookie. Calories: 198.5/99.3 • Total Fat: 9.9. g/4.9 g • Saturated Fat: 4 g/2 g • Protein: 4.9g/2.5 g • Carbohydrates: 26.1 g/13 g • Fiber: 3.3 g/1.7 g • Sugar: 11 g/5.5 g • Vitamin C: 2.8 mg/1.4 mg • Calcium: 25.8 mg/12.9 mg • Iron 1.1 mg/0.5 mg • Sodium: 96.9 mg/48.4 mg • Zinc: 0.6/0.3 mg • Provides ⅛ carbohydrate serving, ⅛ protein serving, and ⅛ fruit serving for children 1 to 3 years.

Red, White, and Blueberry Overnight Oats

Dina, Anthony, and Janet are always struggling to provide a nutritious breakfast for themselves and their toddlers on rushed days when they have to get their kids to school and themselves to work early in the morning. Overnight oats provide the perfect solution. Their children love preparing their breakfast the night before; pouring the ingredients in the jar, picking out the fruits they want, and having fun shaking all the ingredients together. A great way to get toddlers involved in their own nutrition (and busy parents out the door in the morning)! | MAKES 1 SERVING, ABOUT 1 CUP

½ cup rolled oats (not quick cooking or instant)

¼ cup skim milk (may substitute whole, 2%, or almond for adults, or whole for toddlers under 2 years)

1 teaspoon chia seeds

¼ teaspoon of cinnamon

¼ cup plain low-fat yogurt (full-fat for toddlers under 2 years)

1 teaspoon vanilla extract

1½ teaspoons of honey

¼ cup strawberries, diced

¼ cup blueberries, diced

2 tablespoons sliced toasted almonds (ground for toddlers) (see Note)

Prep time: 5 minutes

Excellent source for lactating moms of fiber, vitamins B$_{12}$ and C, calcium, iron, and omega 3 fatty acids.

Good source for lactating moms of protein, vitamin E, and zinc.

In a jar or bowl, mix together the oats, milk, chia seeds, cinnamon, yogurt, vanilla, and honey until thoroughly combined. Add the strawberries and blueberries on top and cover the container. Place the oats in the refrigerator overnight. In the morning, stir the oats with the berries and sprinkle with toasted almonds. Refrigerate for up to 2 days.

Note

We added less milk to make a thicker consistency, but feel free to add more milk to make the oats a thinner consistency. You can also adjust the ingredients to your taste—add less cinnamon, use vanilla yogurt instead of using vanilla extract with plain yogurt, maple syrup instead of honey, different fruit combinations like bananas, blueberries, mangoes, or pineapples, or add in peanut butter and chocolate. The possibilities are endless!

To toast almonds, preheat oven to 350°F. Spread almonds in a single layer on a shallow baking dish or cookie sheet. Place in the oven for 5-10 minutes until they begin to turn a light golden brown. Keep an eye on them closely so they do not burn.

NUTRIENTS PER SERVING FOR ADULTS/TODDLERS PREPARED WITH WHOLE MILK AND FULL FAT YOGURT: 1 serving: 1 cup/½ cup. Calories: 372.5/193.9 • Total Fat: 11 g/7 g • Saturated Fat: 1.7 g/1.7 g • Protein: 13.9 g/6.3 g • Carbohydrates: 56.6 g/27.5 g • Fiber: 8.7 g/4.4 g • Sugar: 23.7 g/11.1 g • Vitamin B$_{12}$: 0.7 mcg/0.3 mcg • Vitamin C: 28.6 mg/14.2 mg • Vitamin E: 3.4 mg/1.7 mg • Calcium: 255.7 mg/106 mg • Iron: 2.9 mg/1.5 mg • Omega 3 fatty acids: 0.7 g/0.4 g • Sodium: 70.9 mg/28.4 mg • Zinc: 1.5 mg/0.6 mg • **Provides 1 carbohydrate serving, ½ protein serving, ¼ dairy serving, and ¼ fruit serving for children 1 to 3 years.**

Chapter Two

~~~~~~~~~~~~~~~~~~~~~~

4 to 6 Months

In chapter two, we discuss the new challenge of introducing complementary foods and answer questions that commonly come up at this early stage of infant feeding. We discuss when, how, and what to feed your baby, tips on baby food preparation, how to tell if a baby is having a serious or not so-serious reaction to a new food, and advise on how to deal with persistent acid reflux and constipation. We end with recipes for first baby foods that are also designed to do double duty—they can be easily transformed into a snack or meal for an older toddler or hungry parent.

Expected Developmental Milestones

Congratulations! You have survived many sleepless nights with a newborn, and by 4 months your little one has turned into a more playful, interactive baby! Gross motor skills now include sitting with support, rolling front to back (4 to 6 months) and back to front (6 to 7 months), bearing weight on their forearms, pushing up to their elbows during tummy time (they actually might even like tummy time now), and bringing their hands together. They are now developing the key skills needed to begin eating solid foods, such as good head control, bringing their hands to their mouths, and showing interest in food by reaching for food on your plate, opening their mouths when a spoon approaches, and closing their mouths and turning away when they are full. Social and language development bring laughter, orientation to voices, and liking to look around (you may notice your baby getting easily distracted when feeding).

Your baby is on a schedule now and many babies are able to sleep through the night (ten to twelve hours of uninterrupted sleep without waking up for middle-of-the-night feedings!) and have a more predictable schedule of feeding, napping, and sleeping. At 6 months, in addition to rolling over, babies' motor skills may include rocking back and forth on their hands and knees to get ready for crawling (some babies, however, may skip crawling), discovering their feet and loving putting them in their mouth, and sitting while leaning forward on their arms (known as tripoding). Babies may reach and grasp objects in a rake-like fashion and transfer objects between hands. Your baby's language skills start to take off, with babbling, razzes, and squeals of delight, and you will be able to have a good back-and-forth social interaction with them.

If you have questions about your child's general development or readiness to start solids, please speak to your pediatrician to address your concerns. Make sure to discuss when to start solids at your child's 4-month health care visit.

Developmental Milestones for 4–6 Months

AGE	MOTOR AND VISUAL SKILLS	SOCIAL SKILLS	COGNITIVE/ LANGUAGE
4 months	Sits with support, rolls front to back (4–6 months), bears weight on forearms during tummy time, reaches with arms, brings hands together and objects to mouth. Range of vision is several feet.	Laughs, orients to voices, and likes to look around.	Responds to tone in caregiver's voice.
6 months	Rolls both ways (6–7 months), rocks back and forth on hands and knees to get ready for crawling, discovers feet and loves putting them in mouth, sits while leaning forward with support of arms (tripoding). Reaches and grasps objects in a rake-like fashion, can reach with one hand, and transfers objects between hands.	Has a good back and forth social interaction with caregiver.	Makes a variety of sounds, babbles, razzes, and squeals.

Adapted from The Harriet Lane Handbook, *17th Edition, and* AAP Caring for Your Baby and Young Child, Birth to Age 5, *4th Edition.*

FEEDING SKILLS

Tongue thrust and rooting reflex fade, making spoon feeding possible, good head control, shows interest in food, brings hands to mouth, reaches for food on caregiver's plate, opens mouth when a spoon comes near, makes up-and-down chewing motion, is able to transfer food from front to back of mouth, closes mouth when full and turns away, may start to drink from sippy cup at 6 months with help from caregiver (with variable success!)

Basic Nutritional Guidelines

There is so much confusing information available to parents on the Internet, along with differing opinions from family and friends on when, how, and what to feed your baby, that it is often hard to know what advice is best to follow. This section begins with a typical menu and how to introduce solid foods. We then discuss special diets, the potential health dangers of drinking unpasteurized milk, the differences between yogurt and whole milk, and whether to give babies extra water or juice. We end the section with our recommendations for introducing sippy, straw, and open cups.

Typical Menu for 4 to 6 Months

Here are some general feeding guidelines from 4 to 6 months. Each day is divided into six different time frames, but remember, these are just guidelines. We mention throughout this book that it is always best to go by your baby's hunger cues, and never force-feed, but also do not be afraid to give more if your baby is hungry.

Range of Calories per Day	
AGE	CALORIES PER DAY*
4–6 Months	Males: 548–645
	Females: 508–593

This range of calories is an estimate based on the average child. Your child may require more or less calories.

Adapted from USDA Food and Nutrition Service's Infant Nutrition and Feeding Guide for use in the WIC and CSF Programs.

Early Morning: Breastfeeding or 4 to 6 ounces breast milk or formula

Breakfast: Breastfeeding or 1 to 2 tablespoons of cereal plus 1 to 2 tablespoons stage 1 fruit, veggie, meat, or poultry

Mid-morning: Breastfeeding or 4 to 6 ounces breast milk or formula

Lunch: Breastfeeding or 4 to 6 ounces breast milk or formula

Late afternoon: Breastfeeding or 4 to 6 ounces breast milk or formula

Bedtime: Breastfeeding or 4 to 6 ounces breast milk or formula

Totals:

Milk intake: 4 to 6 feeds; approximately 26 to 36 ounces per day

Grains: up to 1 serving iron-fortified cereal (1 serving: 1 to 2 tablespoons)

Fruits and vegetables: up to 1 serving of stage 1 (1 serving: 1 to 2 tablespoons)

Proteins: up to 1 serving of stage 1 (1 serving: 1 to 2 tablespoons)

The above menu is based on babies who started complementary foods closer to 6 months. If your baby started solids closer to 4 months, he/she may already be eating solids twice a day, as seen in the menu for 7-month-olds on page 107.

> **What are stage 1 and 2 foods?**
> Stage 1 foods are single ingredient, highly pureed fruits, vegetables, or meats with a smooth texture and thin consistency. Stage 2 foods are thicker and are either single ingredient or simple combination foods. Stage 3 foods are bite-sized beginner finger foods.

Introduction of Solid Foods

Your little baby is growing up fast! Although breast milk or formula will continue to be the main source of nutrition at this stage, many babies will show obvious interest in what you are eating, too. This is an exciting time of many firsts for you and your child—watching him/her enjoy a first taste of solid food is one of those moments you will always treasure. This section includes topics such as how to know when your baby is ready to start solid foods, what are good foods to introduce first, foods not to give, how to store homemade baby food, and will end with a discussion on the nutritional concerns associated with special diets.

What are the signs that my baby is ready to start complementary food?

Signs that your baby is ready to start solid or complementary foods include good head control and the ability to sit with some support, becoming unsatisfied after feeding, shortened intervals between feedings of breast milk or formula, and giving cues that they are finished feeding such as turning their heads when they are done. When your baby is staring you down and grabbing food from your plate, it is time to start solids!

When do I start solids?

This is an area with a bit of debate. The American Academy of Pediatrics (AAP) Section on Breastfeeding and the World Health Organization recommend exclusive breastfeeding until 6 months of age. The AAP Committee on Nutrition recommends that complementary foods, in developed countries, can be introduced between 4 to 6 months of age. Likewise, the USDA states that children are developmentally ready to start solids between 4 to 6 months. The European Society for Pediatric Gastroenterology, Hepatology, and Nutrition recommends that exclusive breastfeeding for about 6 months is desirable but complementary feeding should be introduced no earlier than 17 weeks and no later than 26 weeks of age. In addition, since there is no evidence that suggests food allergy can be prevented by delaying solid food introduction beyond 4 to 6 months, the American Academy of Allergy, Asthma and Immunology recommends 4 to 6 months of age as the right time for introduction of solids. With all this said, most pediatricians will recommend starting solids between 4 and 6 months, depending on a baby's readiness.

We recommend that babies who are exclusively breastfed start solids at 6 months old, or as early as 4 months if they are showing interest. Infants using formula may start as early as 4 months, if they are developmentally ready. A baby's intestines are mature enough to handle solids during this time. A reflex known as the extrusion reflex, in which a baby pushes food out of his/her mouth instead of swallowing the food, will diminish at this age. Starting solids before 4 months in a baby who isn't developmentally ready can interfere with a baby getting all the adequate nutrition provided through breast milk or formula. Introducing solid foods too early has also been linked to obesity. Starting solids by six months helps with oral-motor development and is also important to provide your baby with all the nutrition needed to ensure proper growth, including sufficient amounts of iron and zinc. For example, babies solely drinking whole or breast milk at one year old may become anemic from the lack of iron and the necessary nutrients in their diets (see page 66 for information on iron and zinc). The phrase, "food before one is just for fun" is cute, but not at all true.

Where should my child sit when starting solid foods?

Since your baby will have good head control and will be able to sit with some support, you can begin feeding with your child sitting in a baby seat or on a caregiver's lap, and when he/she can sit well, in a high chair. We do not recommend feeding your baby lying down or in a horizontal position as this can lead to gagging on food and may exacerbate symptoms of gastroesophageal reflux.

How do I introduce solid foods?

There are no strict rules on the best order to give pureed foods to your baby and you should just have fun with it—there are many correct ways to do it. We still recommend, however, giving each new food for three to five days before moving on to the next new food. If an allergic reaction occurs, it will then be easy to identify the culprit. It is also helpful to give the new food in the morning, either before or about an hour after breast milk or formula, when babies are alert and eager to eat. Babies can also be more easily observed for any allergies during the daytime. If you give the new food before bedtime, you risk missing a reaction, and your baby may also be more tired, cranky, and therefore less interested in trying new things.

Remember, when first starting out, breast milk or formula is still going to be the main source of nutrition; solid foods are considered complementary foods and the amount of milk intake usually remains the same at this time. As babies take more and more solids, they will gradually and naturally reduce their milk intake. We often start with solid foods once a day for about four weeks, then twice a day for another month, and then three times a day, so by about eight to nine months most babies will be on solid foods three times a day. This is a general guideline, however, and if your baby seems to be hungry or if your pediatrician suggests, you may move to three solid meals per day at a quicker pace. One-year-olds who are breastfeeding should continue to breastfeed as long as mom and child desire. They can also wean to whole milk, or a combination of the two. Formula-fed infants may also transition to whole milk at one year. One-year-old babies should drink sixteen to a maximum of twenty-four ounces of milk per day (less is fine if they are getting other sources of calcium), eat three meals per day, plus healthy snacks in between.

What foods are good to start with and how much should my child be eating at each meal?

Many pediatricians are still traditional and recommend starting with baby cereal, which is easy to digest and fortified with iron and vitamins, since babies begin to lose their maternal iron stores around 6 months old. Other pediatricians will advise to start with fruits first since babies are naturally drawn to sweet foods, some will recommend vegetables first so babies won't only gravitate toward sweet foods, and still other pediatricians recommend meats first for added iron and zinc. As you can see, little evidence exists that

Top Nine Allergenic Foods

- **Eggs**
- **Fish**
- **Milk**
- **Peanuts**
- **Sesame seeds**
- **Shellfish**
- **Soy**
- **Tree nuts** such as almonds, cashews, chestnuts, pecans, and walnuts
- **Wheat**

the order for introducing solid foods matters and just because you gave your baby vegetables first does not mean your child will be a lifelong veggie lover and never want a sweet! It is more important to offer a variety of fruits, vegetables, and meats in any order to get your baby used to different tastes. Since some foods tend to constipate babies while others have more of a laxative effect, it is also a good idea to give a balance of these foods and adjust them according to your baby's bowel habits.

If you decide to start with cereal (we personally like infant oatmeal best), mix one tablespoon of cereal with four or five tablespoons of formula or breast milk, until the mixture is runny and thin, or a souplike consistency. You *can* start, however, with any stage 1 food. If making your own baby food, the puree should start off similar to the thin consistency of stage 1 foods.

Initially, the serving size at this age is typically one to two tablespoons and will increase with age. You can spoon-feed your baby as much of the prepared cereal or stage 1 puree as he/she wants. Never put food in your baby's bottle, unless your baby has acid reflux and you have been instructed by your doctor to mix cereal in the bottle. Be respectful of your baby's desire to eat when he/she is hungry and stop when your baby is full; don't use distractions like televisions or tablets as your baby may eat more even when full. Always go by your baby's cues and never force-feed, but do not be afraid to give more if your baby still looks hungry. This will help your baby know when he/she is hungry and stop when he/she is full, and will help your baby develop healthy eating habits when your baby is later able to self-feed. Ways babies will show you that they are done eating include turning their head, keeping their mouth closed when offered more, and losing interest in feeding. If your baby is not interested in solid feeding, then take a break and wait a few days before starting again. Remember, feeding is supposed to be fun and messy, but not stressful!

When your baby has gotten the hang of eating the purees that are thinner in consistency, he/she will be ready for stage 2 foods. After six months, when a few first foods have been added into your baby's diet, we recommend introducing the more highly allergenic foods including whole milk yogurt, whole Greek yogurt, low mercury fish, and peanut and nut butters (see chart, opposite, and page 86).

When your baby is about 8 or 9 months old and has developed an immature grasp and is sitting well alone, he/she will be then be ready for stage 3 foods, which are chunkier in texture, and finger foods.

Giving Yogurt To Your Baby

Which yogurt you give your baby comes down to reading labels! Although many of the flavored baby yogurts have added sugar in them (beyond the natural sugar, lactose, found in dairy) or juice rather than just fruit, they often also have added vitamin D in them, too. Many adult plain whole milk yogurts lack this added vitamin D. If your child is not receiving an adequate amount of vitamin D, we suggest using a plain baby yogurt without added sugar and adding your own fruits or veggies to it. If you use a yogurt without added vitamin D (the large adult yogurt containers are often much more economical!), make sure there are other adequate sources of vitamin D in your child's diet.

In addition, Greek yogurt typically contains more fat and protein and less sugar than the whole milk equivalent. If your child is allergic to milk, however, your pediatrician may recommend delaying the introduction of milk products until a later age and may recommend other alternatives including coconut or soy yogurt. Please check with your pediatrician as these products may also have lower nutritional content.

Iron, Zinc, and Your Baby

Iron and zinc are essential nutrients for all healthy full-term infants. Most full-term infants are born with adequate iron stores, which is depleted at around 4 to 6 months old. Since breast milk is low in iron, iron-fortified infant cereals or pureed meats are especially important for breastfed infants. Likewise, zinc, which is involved in supporting our immune system, skin healing, and our senses of smell and taste, is obtained from breast milk, which is an adequate source of zinc until 6 months old. After 6 months, breast milk does not provide all the zinc a baby needs, so babies should be provided additional zinc through complementary food (such as meat and fortified infant cereal). Of note, infant formulas are fortified with iron and zinc.

Constipating and Laxative Foods

Constipating foods include rice cereal, potatoes, bananas, and apple-sauce. Laxative foods include those that begin with the letter "P," such as prunes, pears, peaches, plums, papayas, and aPricots.

Timing of Introduction of Solid Food

AGE	FOOD
4–6 months	Baby cereals including rice and oatmeal, stage 1 or single ingredient fruits, veggies, meats, or poultry
6–8 months	Baby cereals including barley and wheat (6 months), stage 2 or combination foods with thicker textures when ready, full-fat yogurt, soy protein (tofu), pureed or well-mashed beans, peanut butter (6–8 months, can be mixed with yogurt or a puree so not a choking hazard), tree nut butter (7–9 months after other allergenic foods tolerated, can also be mixed with yogurt or a puree so not a choking hazard), pureed eggs or low-mercury fish/shellfish (though we find that babies often prefer to eat these as finger foods)
8–12 months	Stage 3 finger foods, small pieces of soft cheese, meat, poultry, low-mercury fish, scrambled eggs, peanut and tree nut butters (on cracker as thin smear after other allergenic foods)
1 year+	Whole milk, honey, anything you are eating (excluding choking hazards)

See individual chapters for more food examples.

Should I avoid giving my baby highly allergic foods?

For years parents were told to avoid giving babies "highly" allergenic foods like peanut butter, eggs, and shellfish until after a year of age. The AAP, however, now believes that there is not enough convincing evidence to suggest delaying the introduction of these highly allergenic foods as a strategy to reduce the risk of developing a food allergy. There is emerging evidence suggesting that delay of introduction to milk, egg, wheat, and peanut may increase the risk of these food allergies and the risk of other allergic conditions, such as eczema. At this point, based on current evidence, for a child who is not at high risk for developing food allergies, allergists suggest that you start adding the more allergenic foods by 12 months (see page 86). If your child is at a higher risk for food allergies, such as having a sibling or parent with food allergies, persistent moderate to severe eczema, or allergies to other foods already introduced, discussion with your child's pediatrician or evaluation by an allergist may be helpful to determine if and when it is safe to start feeding your baby all allergenic foods.

Do I have to start with rice cereal?

There is a bit of controversy about giving rice cereal after the FDA found varying amounts of arsenic in rice products. Rice contains high levels of inorganic arsenic, which is particularly true for rice bran. Further research is needed to assess the actual long-term impact of arsenic. Currently, the AAP advises that babies consume a well-balanced diet, including rice along with different grains such as oat, barley, wheat, and maize. This can be difficult for children with food allergies and celiac disease where arsenic intake is estimated to be higher due to diet limitations and dependence on rice.

With so many good baby food choices, cereal does not have be the first food introduced. If you do decide to introduce grains, we personally recommend to

Arsenic

Arsenic can be found naturally in water, air, food, and soil or can be the result of contamination from human actions, such as mining and using pesticides containing arsenic. Arsenic occurs in two forms. Inorganic arsenic is thought to be harmful and associated with negative health effects, while organic is harmless. Arsenic can be present in many foods because it can be absorbed from the soil and water. Rice can take up arsenic from soil and water more easily than other foods.

start with oatmeal. If you give your child rice cereal, we recommend offering up to one serving of rice per day. In reality, you can move on to a new food in three to five days, so giving rice cereal should not be a point of stress.

Should I only be giving my baby superfoods?

Books, magazines, television, and other media often use the term "superfood." Frankly, the term can lead parents into thinking that these foods are absolutely essential for a child to be eating, which can be stressful if the child refuses to eat that particular food. There is no one "it" food or list of foods that cures all ailments. Yes, the usual list of "it" superfoods are healthy (such as avocado, kale, quinoa, blueberries), but as we will say throughout this book, it is always best to eat a wide variety of fruits, vegetables, whole grains, dairy, lean meat, and fish (if your diet permits), and not only to concentrate on a small list of foods that are reportedly a must to eat.

Why can I give my baby yogurt but not whole milk?

Whole milk does not contain as many nutrients as breast milk or formula and is harder for babies to digest. If babies were to drink large volumes of whole milk, it could fill them up so they are not eating more nutritious foods. It can also lead to iron-deficiency anemia because it is lower in iron, may fill children up so they are not eating more iron-rich foods, and can also irritate the stomach lining, causing a microscopic gastrointestinal bleed in children under one year of age. This gastrointestinal response typically resolves by 12 months old.

Yogurt or cheese is easier to digest due to the fermentation process and is not consumed in such large quantities that would interfere with your baby eating other nutritious foods. If your baby does not have a cow's milk protein allergy, and if they have tolerated a few first foods, you can discuss with your pediatrician about starting plain whole milk yogurt or Greek yogurt at 6 months.

Are there any foods that I should not give my baby?

There are some foods that you should not feed your child at this age. For example, honey, foods containing honey (like honey-sweetened cereals or graham crackers), and possibly light and dark corn syrups, cannot be given before one year of life due to the risk of botulism. Babies should also not be eating unpasteurized dairy or juices, undercooked fish, meat, egg, or poultry, or home-canned foods, which could potentially be contaminated with bacteria. Babies should also not be drinking whole milk under 1 year of age.

In addition, if there is a strong family history of food allergies, or if your baby has a history of severe allergic disease or has severe eczema that is hard to treat, it is best to ask your pediatrician for further guidance before giving a food that can potentially cause an allergic reaction in your baby.

Botulism

Infant botulism occurs predominantly in babies less than 6 months old when ingested spores of a bacteria called *Clostridium botulinum* multiply and produce its toxin in the baby's intestine. Symptoms of botulism include constipation, decreased movement, poor feeding, decreased tone, weak cry, and loss of developmental milestones such as head control. According to the CDC, there are approximately one hundred cases of infantile botulism annually in the United States. On average, it occurs between 4 to 5 months of age. In addition to honey, it is also best to avoid light and dark corn syrups before 1 year old, because they may contain *Clostridium botulinum* spores.

Can I feed my baby unpasteurized milk?

Definitely not! Consuming unpasteurized milk and milk products poses risks to pregnant women and infants. According to the CDC, unpasteurized milk is 150 times more likely to lead to illness and results in 13 times more hospitalizations than sicknesses caused by pasteurized dairy. Pasteurization raises the temperature of milk to at least 161°F for more than fifteen seconds followed by rapid cooling. This process eliminates bacteria such as *Listeria, Campylobacter, Salmonella, Brucella,* and *E-coli* that may lead to serious life-threatening illnesses such as meningitis and blood-borne and diarrheal infections in infants.

Additional Sources of Unpasteurized Foods and Drinks

Certain types of cheese (like brie or feta) or juice (such as juices from farmers' markets or local juice bars) may be unpasteurized. Check labels carefully! If you can not determine if the product has been pasteurized, it is best not to serve it.

Does my baby need extra water throughout the day?

Babies do not need water since they are getting all the nutrients and hydration they need from breast milk or formula even on a hot day. Breast milk and formula is comprised of approximately 88 percent water. The addition of extra water can fill an infant's stomach up so that the infant is not taking as much milk as required. After 6 months, when solid foods are introduced, water in a sippy cup can also be added to the baby's diet, at approximately 4 ounces in a day. After a year, when we want to limit the amount of whole milk to 16 to 24 ounces, if your baby is growing well, they can drink water with meals or when thirsty at other times.

Can I give my baby juice?

Babies and children typically never need juice. Though prune and pear juice may be used to treat occasional constipation, regular use of juice is not recommended. Juice is full of empty calories, can lead to excess weight gain, and fills your baby up so he/she won't eat more nutritious foods. Although juice contains fruit, the majority of the fiber has been eliminated. If you do decide to give juice, do so after 6 months of age, with only 100 percent fruit juice. Offer it in a cup and not in a bottle, and in a limited amount. According to the AAP, children over 1 year of age may drink up to four to six ounces of juice per day.

What foods may cause flatulence?

All children will pass gas and this is normal. It does not necessarily mean that your child is having a negative reaction to food. Gas is caused by swallowed air and by normal bacteria in your child's intestines in response to foods that are more complex to digest. Every child will react to food differently. Since children eat very frequently, it is hard to know what the exact cause of the gas may be. Though the foods listed below may cause flatulence, they also are quite nutritious and should not be avoided. Over time your child can adapt to these foods as the body adjusts to breaking it down.

Here is a list of grains, fruits, and veggies that commonly lead to increased gas in children (and adults!):

Grains: bran, oatmeal, wheat

Vegetables: asparagus, broccoli, Brussels sprouts, cabbage, cauliflower, corn, onions

Fruits: apricots, prunes, peaches, pears, plums, citrus fruits

When can I introduce a sippy cup or a straw cup?

You can start offering a few ounces of water (much less messy when spilled than milk) in a sippy cup at 6 months old. There are many types of options, such as hard or soft spouts, spouts that resemble nipples, and cups with or without handles. It might be hard at first to transition, so you can help your baby by lifting the cup together and helping place it in his/her mouth. For some babies it takes a little bit of practice, while others may refuse drinking from the sippy cup. If your baby is refusing to drink from the cup, make sure that the valve system in the cup isn't making it too hard to draw out the water. After your baby gets the hang of a sippy cup, you can begin transitioning to a straw cup at around 1 year old, or sooner if your baby is ready. Switching quickly off the sippy cup comes from controversy on whether the use of sippy cups might prevent the use of muscles needed for speech development, since children may push out their tongue and suck on the sippy cup like they do on a bottle or pacifier.

The goal is to be off the bottle by around 15 months, and to begin using an open cup, ideally by 2 years old or sooner (we know this may seem easier said than done). After your baby gets the hang of drinking water from a straw cup, you can start offering milk in it. Many babies might push away milk offered in a straw cup since they are used to the familiar bottle or breast. We recommend going cold turkey and removing bottles from the house. If your baby is having a hard time, try warming the milk or transitioning off one of the midday bottles first, followed by the morning, and lastly the night. Remember that sippy cups, straw cups, and bottles should never be left in the mouth while the baby is sleeping in the crib. This can lead to cavities.

Bottle weaning might seem like a daunting task, but it is much easier to say ba-bye to the ba-ba sooner rather than later.

Are there any other foods I should consider not giving my baby?

Citrus and acidic fruits like oranges, tomatoes, and lemons are not a definite no-no, but too much may lead to a skin rash or may exacerbate acid reflux symptoms. You may choose to keep these in limited quantities in the diet, if your baby is experiencing any unwanted effects from them.

By the same token, you do not have to eliminate foods that create excess gas, but if you think your child is sensitive to these foods, you can limit these foods as well.

Preparing Your Own Baby Food

Ready to start making homemade baby food? If you are anything like Dina and Anthony and love to cook but have no special training in cooking, we thought it would be helpful to discuss the four steps of food handling, including cooking temperatures, and what you need to get started making baby food. Spoiler alert—nothing special is needed!

Handling food properly to prevent food-borne illnesses is essential when preparing baby food. Proper food handling basically boils down to four steps:

1. Wash your hands, cooking surfaces, and utensils thoroughly. Properly clean all the surfaces coming in contact with your food before you begin to prepare your meal. Wash your hands with warm soapy water for at least twenty seconds before handling food or eating.

2. Don't cross-contaminate. Make sure to clean your cooking utensils and mixing bowls with hot soapy water thoroughly in between contact with foods such as raw eggs, chicken, beef, and fish.

3. Cook to the appropriate temperature and know your proper temperatures for safe consumption (see chart, opposite). Many foodborne illnesses result from consuming raw poultry, meat, and fish. Buy a meat and poultry thermometer to prevent any mistakes and measure the temperature of meat before removing it from heat.

4. Refrigerate foods. When you get home from the grocery store, make sure to store food within two hours, in a refrigerator that is set at 40°F (4.4°C) or below or in a freezer that is at 0°F (-17.7°C) or below. If thawing previously frozen poultry, fish, or meat, it is best to do so on the bottom shelf of the refrigerator so that drippings don't contaminate other foods.

What do I need to make my own food?

To start making your own baby food, the most valuable tool you will need is something to help mash and puree the food. There are a variety of gadgets available for this purpose, including a regular or an immersion blender, potato masher, food mill, food processor, or specialized baby food maker. We personally made our own baby food with an immersion blender, regular blender, or food processor, since we already had these in our homes. Other than a means to puree food, a few pots, pans, baby soft-tipped spoons, and ice cube trays for freezing and storage, nothing special is needed to get started!

Proper Cooking Temperatures for Meat, Poultry, and Fish

TYPE OF FOOD	MINIMAL INTERNAL TEMPERATURE
Beef, pork, lamb, veal, steaks, chops, and roasts	145°F (62.8°C)
Ground meats	160°F (71.1°C)
Poultry	165°F (73.9°C)
Fish and shellfish	145°F (62.8°C)

Are there any foods that I shouldn't make on my own?

Some parents wonder if they should avoid vegetables that are grown in soil and may contain nitrates. Examples of vegetables that may contain higher amounts of nitrates include beets, carrots, squash, spinach, collard greens, green beans, broccoli, and other root vegetables. Nitrates can be potentially harmful when converted by bacteria to nitrites, which can lead to a rare form of anemia called methemoglobinemia, commonly known as blue baby syndrome. Though the overall risk is very low, it is important to limit exposure to nitrites. The majority of cases are usually associated with high nitrate levels found in contaminated well water. Normal nitrate levels are less than ten parts per million. If you are using well water, we recommend either using bottled water or having your well water tested for nitrates. As infants under 3 months of age are more susceptible to methemoglobinemia, the AAP recommends that high nitrate vegetables be avoided before 3 months of age, which is easy to follow since we do not introduce solid foods to babies before 4 to 6 months of age. We recommend to play it safe and to introduce homemade versions of these vegetables after your child is 6 months old, since by this time their stomach acid should protect them and limit the risk of nitrate exposure.

Homemade Purees and High-Nitrate Foods

Pureeing releases an enzyme that increases the conversion of nitrates to nitrites in vegetables. Therefore, at this age, purees of these vegetables should be consumed within twenty-four hours or be frozen when eating is delayed for more than twenty-four hours, since freezing blocks nitrites from accumulating.

Baby Food Storage Time		
SOLIDS (OPENED OR HOMEMADE)	REFRIGERATOR	FREEZER
Strained fruits and vegetables	2 days	1 month
High-nitrate vegetable purees	1 day	1 month
Strained meats, poultry, fish, and eggs	1 day	1 month

Adapted from the FDA and USDA

How long does baby food last?

According to the FDA, store-purchased strained fruits and veggies can be refrigerated for two to three days, meats and eggs for one day, meat and veggie combos for one to two days, and homemade baby foods for one to two days (except for homemade high-nitrate vegetables, which should be used within twenty-four hours). Always check the jar, tub, or pouch of baby food, however, since many of the containers will say to discard after two days, while the pouches will state to discard after twenty-four hours. Reading labels is important! When feeding your baby food from a jar, it is best to remove the portion of food your baby is going to eat and place it in a separate container. If you feed directly from the baby jar, you risk contaminating the jar with bacteria from your baby's mouth. Any food left over from a jar you directly fed from should be thrown out and not saved for later use.

Special Diets

Families often try non-conventional diets for a variety of reasons, including an effort to boost health or lose weight, and some parents consider including their children in these dietary practices. It's important to be aware of the potential health dangers and nutritional limitations of some of these fad diets.

What is baby-led weaning and is it recommended over the "traditional" approach of starting solids?

Baby-led weaning (BLW) is defined as an alternative method of starting solids in which babies over 6 months are introduced to solid foods by feeding themselves pieces of food at the family meal-time rather than being spoon-fed purees. In baby-led weaning, the parent offers pieces of whole food, making

> ## Choking in Babies
> We have seen babies in our office who have had severe difficulty breathing, and have required surgery to remove bits of food from their airway that they have choked on. Babies *can definitely* choke; as parents ourselves, witnessing a baby in any distress is always difficult. It has led us to stick with the traditional way we have always fed babies: starting with purees and, when developmentally ready, moving on to thicker textures and finger foods. This more traditional way leads to adventurous eaters as well, and in a manner we feel is more in line with their level of development.

purees and spoon feeding unnecessary, and the baby decides what and how much to eat and how long it will take to do so. It is thought that this method leads to babies regulating the way they eat and to healthier body weights and adventurous eaters.

We cannot comfortably recommend baby-led weaning due to the lack of research and large-scale studies supporting the method. We have several concerns with this diet, foremost of which is the risk of choking. In addition, not all babies will have the motor skills necessary for self-feeding and the ability to take in enough food to meet their nutritional requirements. Babies lose their maternal iron stores at around 6 months of age and require iron-rich foods, such as iron-fortified cereals and meats. It is uncertain if babies who follow BLW will consume sufficient amounts of iron. Also, salt and sugar intake may be a concern if babies are given highly salted and sugary foods that the family is eating. Lastly, exposure to family meals with multiple ingredients may also make it difficult to identify or isolate an allergen, if an allergic reaction to a dish with several new food ingredients occurs. With all this said, if you feel this diet meets your family's needs, we suggest developing a diet plan with the help of your pediatrician.

If I want to raise my baby as a vegetarian, what do I need to know?
According to the AAP, vegetarian diets can meet the needs of children if planned out carefully. There is even some evidence that vegetarian diets may be higher in fiber, and lower in cholesterol than diets that include meat. However, it becomes more difficult to ensure that all nutritional needs are being met if vegetarian diets are very restrictive and eliminate multiple food groups, especially if they are vegan.

There are a few major nutritional concerns with different types of vegetarian diets.

Protein: Vegetarians with limited or no animal food sources in their diet will have to monitor their intake of protein sources. Animal-based foods like meats, eggs, and dairy products contain complete proteins. Non-animal-based proteins should come from multiple sources to provide a varied mixture of amino acids (the building blocks of proteins). For example, one might combine whole-wheat cereals with legumes like beans, peanuts, or soy, or with seeds like quinoa, sunflower, or chia.

Vitamins and Minerals: With a meat-free and seafood-free diet, vegetarians may be at risk of consuming inadequate amounts of zinc, iron, and other minerals mainly found in these animal-based products. When dairy is eliminated from the diet, intake of calcium and vitamins B_{12} and D may be insufficient. For vegetarians and vegans, who eliminate whole food groups, it may be necessary to provide specific foods fortified with added vitamin B_{12}, zinc, and minerals (such as fortified nondairy beverages, or fortified breakfast cereals), use a complete multivitamin supplement, and possibly additional calcium and vitamin D supplements.

As with any diet where whole food groups are eliminated, total fat and total calorie intake may also be inadequate. With all this said, we do believe vegetarian diets can be a healthy option for young children, but if you decide to follow a vegan diet for your child, we highly advise reviewing your child's diet with your pediatrician and with a registered dietitian to ensure that he or she is getting all the nutrients needed for proper growth and development.

Common Classifications of Vegetarian Diets

NAME	DIET INCLUDES
Lacto-ovo-vegetarian	Plant-based food, dairy products, and eggs
Lacto-vegetarian	Plant-based food and dairy products
Vegan	Plant-based food only; no food from any animal sources

Without proper monitoring, restricted diets may result in poor weight gain and nutritional deficiencies.

Is the paleo diet safe for my baby?

The paleo diet is intended to mimic the diet of our hunter and gatherer ancestors. It includes meats, fish, fruits, eggs, nonstarchy vegetables, seeds, and natural oils like olive or coconut. The diet calls for avoiding grains, legumes, soy, fruit juice, iodized salt, highly processed oils, and refined sugars. We do not recommend this diet for children since it may be unsafe as it lacks many dietary sources of carbohydrates that are essential for a growing child. It also may have inadequate amounts of nutrients such as calcium, vitamin D, B vitamins, and other micronutrients like iodine.

What is the raw diet?

A raw diet consists of uncooked foods such as fresh fruits, vegetables, seeds, nuts, and sprouted grains. Some who follow this diet also include raw meats or fish, and raw or unpasteurized milk, yogurt, or cheese. This diet is not recommended for use in children. This diet may lack sufficient protein and micronutrients. A raw diet may provide fiber in amounts well beyond the recommended daily intake of fiber, and it could potentially be difficult for a young child to tolerate due to gas, loose stools, or bloating. If raw meats and unpasteurized dairy products are included, there is a risk of these foods containing harmful bacteria that could cause serious health problems.

My baby is eating more solid foods, should I only make them with organic ingredients?

To date, there are no human studies that directly demonstrate the health benefits of an organic diet or prove it to be nutritionally better than

"DIRTY DOZEN" 2015
(produce with the most amount of pesticides, listed from dirtiest to cleanest)

1. Apple
2. Peach
3. Nectarine
4. Strawberry
5. Grape
6. Celery
7. Spinach
8. Sweet bell pepper
9. Cucumber
10. Cherry tomato
11. Snap pea (imported)
12. Potato

"CLEAN 15" 2015
(produce with the least amount of pesticides)

1. Avocado
2. Sweet corn
3. Pineapple
4. Cabbage
5. Sweet pea, frozen
6. Onion
7. Asparagus
8. Mango
9. Papaya
10. Kiwi
11. Eggplant
12. Grapefruit
13. Cantaloupe
14. Cauliflower
15. Sweet potato

Copyright © Environmental Working Group, www.ewg.org. Reprinted with permission.

conventional foods. The AAP, however, states that organic diets expose people to fewer pesticides associated with human disease and organically raised animals are less likely to be contaminated with drug-resistant bacteria. The more antibiotics an animal receives, the more likely bacteria can become resistant to those drugs and then spread that resistance to human disease.

What do we think? Try to buy organic if you can, but don't stress out about it since the research is still ongoing and the price of organic food can be quite expensive. It is always better to eat a wide variety of conventionally grown fruits and vegetables rather than none at all just to avoid the higher costs of organic foods. Try to wash fruits and vegetables thoroughly, and peel the skin off of conventionally grown high pesticide produce to eliminate even more pesticide residue. We also recommend that you try to avoid buying foods from the Environmental Working Group's (EWG) "Dirty Dozen" list of foods that contain the highest pesticide residue. The EWG is a nonprofit, nonpartisan, environmental health research and advocacy organization, which annually publishes, among other things, the "Dirty Dozen" and the "Clean 15" list of foods (see above).

Expected Growth

From 3 to 6 months, your child should gain an average of 1 ounce every other day or approximately 1 pound per month. This rate is slower than what is expected during the newborn to 3-month period. Children usually double their birth weight by 5 to 6 months of life. Your child will continue to gain approximately $3/4$ inch in length per month and your baby's head circumference should increase by one centimeter per month at this age.

Medical Concerns

The majority of babies will have no issues when starting complementary foods. Some children, however, may develop an allergic reaction to certain foods, an exacerbation of their reflux, or constipation. We discuss these common medical issues as they pertain to your 4 to 6 month old.

Food Allergies

Starting complementary foods is an exciting milestone in a baby's life, but many parents are concerned about how they will know if their child is having an allergic reaction and what to do if an allergic reaction arises. This section discusses the signs of an allergic reaction, what medications to have available, when to call 9-1-1, and our recommendations for when to introduce the more allergenic foods. We end the section with a discussion of food protein–induced enterocolitis.

Why is there a rise in food allergies?

You may not remember anybody having food allergies when you were a child in school. However, your children are very likely to encounter other children with food allergies among their playmates and classmates. This is because the prevalence of food allergies has indeed increased over the past two decades, especially in developed countries, such that food allergies now affect approximately one in thirteen children. As you may know, for some, food allergies can be life-threatening.

Though we do not know exactly why there has been an increase in the number of people affected by food and other allergies, there have been several theories. One of the more interesting theories has been the hygiene hypothesis, which suggests that our increasingly clean, Westernized lifestyle prevents our bodies from coming into contact with microorganisms and bacteria (germs), and that this skews the immune system toward an allergic response. The effect may be most significant for babies and children whose immune systems are still developing and influenced by interactions with things like their environments, pets, diets, illnesses, and siblings. Studies have, in fact, shown fewer allergies among children who grow up on farms, where there is a lot of direct exposure to farm animals. Moreover, we now live in an environment where antibacterial soap cleansers are ubiquitous, food preparation is extremely hygienic, and antibiotics are readily available and often prescribed. It is possible by our overall effort to be clean and avoid infection, that some of the immune benefits of exposure to a less-sanitized environment have been lost.

The hygiene hypothesis does not explain everything about the rise in food allergy prevalence, and the answer is not simply that we get ourselves "dirty," or that your child should lick the stroller wheels. There are other factors that come into play and are actively being investigated, including genetics, environmental pollution, climate change, agriculture, diet patterns, and vitamin deficiencies. There is a complicated interplay of exposures to many features of our modern life that are likely responsible for the rise in allergies as well as other diseases. From ongoing research, we will hopefully have a more complete understanding of these "allergy-provoking" influences.

How do I know if my child is having an allergic reaction to a food?

An allergic reaction may happen when feeding a baby a new food and is most often seen with only a few foods (milk, eggs, soy, wheat, peanuts, tree nuts, sesame, fish, and shellfish). However, this list of foods is not exclusive, and an allergy can occur to almost any food. In general, an allergic reaction does not develop to a food that has already been a regular part of a child's diet.

In infants, it may be difficult to identify an allergic reaction. A 4-month-old baby cannot describe many of the symptoms of an allergic reaction that an older child or adult may be able to verbalize. In general, an allergic reaction will occur while eating or shortly after eating the food allergen. Some allergic reactions are delayed and do not occur until several hours later. It is very unusual, however, for an allergic reaction to start more than six hours after a causative food is eaten.

Allergic reactions are not all the same. The spectrum of allergic reactions ranges from very mild skin reactions or brief gastrointestinal discomfort to severe anaphylaxis. An infant who is having an acute allergic reaction may have almost any of the organ systems of the body involved. There may be just one symptom, or many symptoms may develop all at once. An allergic reaction can also progress to involve more symptoms over time, sometimes slowly and sometimes rather quickly. The following are symptoms that can be seen during an allergic reaction:

Skin: lip or tongue swelling, eyelid swelling, generalized itchiness, skin redness, hives in localized areas or all over the body, or an immediate flare of eczema rash

Digestive: sudden onset of repeated vomiting, or diarrhea

Respiratory: sneezing, coughing, choking, wheezing, or labored breathing

Cardiovascular: pale "white" skin, bluish lips, mouth, or fingers, rapid pulse or weak pulse

Nervous system: irritability, or loss of consciousness

Food Intolerance Versus Food Allergy

Food intolerances are not mediated by the immune system. A food intolerance generally manifests with digestive symptoms (for example, gassiness, bloating, and diarrhea), as seen in lactose intolerance. Food intolerances are not life-threatening and typically do not require emergency intervention. On the other hand, food allergies are immune-mediated and may involve any organ system including the skin, or gastrointestinal, respiratory, cardiovascular, and nervous systems.

Is my baby's rash a sign of a food allergy?

Babies and children develop skin rashes for a lot of different reasons. Not all rashes are signs of an allergic reaction. Babies often develop blotchy rashes, or even hives, on the face where food comes into contact with the skin, and this may just be a topical skin irritation. This is a fairly frequent phenomenon with acidic foods like tomatoes and citrus fruits, as well as berries, and should generally not deter you from trying these particular foods again. If you think your child is having a contact reaction to the food, you may place moisturizer on your child's face to prevent the food from directly contacting your child's skin. In addition, if the food can be eaten in a different form without causing a reaction, such as when your child's skin turns blotchy when eating a blueberry but not while eating a blueberry yogurt, then it is not a true allergy to blueberries. However, if your baby has facial swelling, other organ systems involved, or hives all over the body, and not just where the food came in contact, this may be a true allergic reaction and needs immediate medical attention. If you are uncertain, we recommend talking to your child's pediatrician for guidance.

My baby has eczema. Is this from a food allergy?

The presence of eczema can be a sign that a baby has an allergic disposition, especially if the eczema is persistent, involves a large majority of the skin surface, and is moderate to severe. Sometimes eczema is isolated, but some babies with eczema will go on to develop food allergies, asthma, and environmental allergies later in infancy and childhood.

We do occasionally find that an infant formula or diet, or that maternal diet, if the baby is breastfeeding, can contribute to a baby's eczema. However, eczema is more often *not* directly caused by any of the foods that are already part of the baby's diet. For some infants, we may find that environmental allergens (household pets or dust mites, for example) are major triggers for eczema, while other babies have persistent eczema but have no allergic triggers. Other factors such as skin irritants, viral illnesses, perspiration, heat, cold, and dry ambient air should also be considered, as these can contribute to eczema.

For infants who have persistent eczema (lasting for months) that does not improve with an optimized skin care regimen, especially where there is a family history of food allergies, an allergy evaluation is recommended. We do not recommend changing infant formulas or altering a baby's diet (nor the breastfeeding mother's diet) in an effort to "cure" the eczema without first speaking with a physician.

What medications should I have available when introducing foods?

It is a good idea to always be prepared to treat potential allergic reactions by having children's liquid diphenhydramine (Benadryl) available at home. Liquid diphenhydramine comes in only one strength (12.5 milligrams per teaspoon). There is no special infant version, and although it says on the box not to administer the liquid medication to children under 6 years old, you may give it to younger children under your pediatrician's guidance. Your doctor can instruct you on the appropriate dose, which is based on your child's weight and

A potential allergic reaction can be quite scary for parents to watch! When Julia first started eating solids, Dina noticed she developed a hive on her leg after eating bananas. Dina watched the hive to make sure it didn't spread all over Julia's body and that she didn't develop any signs of a serious reaction like swelling on her tongue, trouble breathing, wheezing, or repetitive vomiting, which would require her to go to a hospital. But the hive quickly resolved on its own and was likely a temporary contact reaction from the banana touching the skin, since Julia continues to enjoy bananas as one of her favorite foods today. The stress of the reaction, however, was mitigated by Dina knowing Julia's Benadryl dose, having the medication on hand in case her daughter needed it, and knowing to call 9-1-1 if any more serious reactions developed.

will increase as your child gains weight. You should know how much to give your child in case an allergic reaction occurs. Although we include a dosing chart for your convenience on page 209, we always recommend first checking with your child's doctor before administering any type of medicine.

Allergy experts recommend the liquid formulation for treating allergic reactions to foods, regardless of age, because it may work faster. Of note, diphenhydramine is an appropriate treatment only for a mild allergic reaction.

What do I do in the event of a severe allergic reaction and how do I know when to call 9-1-1?

Anaphylaxis is a severe and life-threatening situation. If you think your baby or child is having an allergic reaction and appears very ill, call 9-1-1. For instance, if your baby develops difficulty breathing, swelling on the face or tongue, listlessness, becomes unresponsive, or you see symptoms from several of the body systems listed on page 81, call 9-1-1. If you know that your child has a food allergy, it is very important that you speak with your pediatrician or allergist, and educate yourself (and any of your child's caregivers) regarding anaphylaxis.

- You should review the signs and symptoms of anaphylaxis, have an updated and personalized emergency treatment plan, have nonexpired epinephrine autoinjectors (see page 210) available at all times, and make sure that you are trained regarding how and when to use epinephrine.

- You should *not* wait for the ambulance or EMT to arrive before giving epinephrine (remember Benadryl does not treat a severe allergic reaction!).
- It is also important to practice with the epinephrine training devices every three months to ensure that you always know how to use them properly.

Will an allergic food reaction happen after the first or after many exposures?

With classic IgE-mediated food allergies, an allergic reaction may happen with the first taste or bite of a new food, so it is important to watch your baby closely after feeding him or her a new food, particularly those that are known to be highly allergenic (including milk, eggs, soy, wheat, fish, shellfish, peanuts, tree nuts, and sesame). An allergic reaction, however, may not always occur with the first exposure to a new food and may not be apparent until a child has had that new food a few times. This is the reason it is recommended that, with early food introductions, a new food be tried for three to five days before moving on to the next new food, and that multiple new foods not be given for the first time together.

Although there are exceptions, for the most part, food allergies do not develop to foods that have been incorporated as a regular, consistent part of a child's diet. It is possible, though, for an allergy to develop to a food that was only given one time many months or years ago.

Will my child outgrow his/her food allergy?

Many food allergies that appear in infancy do resolve during childhood. Most children who have allergies to milk, eggs, soy, and wheat will eventually outgrow these food allergies and will often do so before school-age. Infants and children who can tolerate milk and egg in baked or well-heated forms tend to outgrow their milk and egg allergies even more rapidly. Allergies to peanuts, tree nuts, and seafood are less likely to be outgrown, but can be transient or resolve in some cases. Children who have known food allergies should be followed regularly by their pediatrician or an allergist, as allergy testing over time (via skin prick tests or IgE levels to foods in the blood) can indicate when and if food allergies are likely to resolve. If your baby or child has been diagnosed with a food allergy, it is important *not* to try feeding the allergenic food at home without first discussing this with your pediatrician and allergist. In many cases, an allergist will suggest a doctor-supervised feeding test (known as an "oral food challenge") in a supervised, controlled office setting to confirm whether a food allergy has been outgrown.

Should I introduce allergenic foods later, such as peanuts, if there is a strong family history of food allergies?

A baby is at a higher risk for developing food allergies if there is a first-degree family member (parent or sibling) who also has food allergies. There is ongoing research about whether the specific foods to which the older sibling or parent is allergic to should be tested first, delayed, or introduced early into the infant's diet.

Specifically for peanuts, there is now evidence that we may be able to prevent peanut allergy from developing in babies who are "at risk" (but not already allergic) by early introduction of peanuts into the diet before 1 year of age. A study published in 2015 showed that for infants who specifically have an egg allergy or eczema, delaying peanut introduction may increase the chance of developing a peanut allergy. We are beginning to recommend that an evaluation specifically for peanut allergy be done between 4 to 8 months for babies with persistent or moderate-to-severe eczema, other food allergies, or a family history of peanut allergy. These babies may have peanut butter introduced between 4 to 11 months of age *after* an allergist states it is safe to do so. Please speak to your pediatrician about these recommendations, and timing for introduction of other allergenic foods, as they are constantly evolving.

When do I introduce the more allergenic foods (eggs, milk, soy, wheat, peanuts, tree nuts, fish, shellfish, and sesame)?

Much of the advice from the past decade regarding the timing of introduction of the top allergenic foods has been more recently revised. It is no longer recommended that you delay introduction of allergenic foods, as there is no good evidence that this prevents the development of food allergies. In fact, it may be counterproductive. Prolonging the time to introducing allergens (when there is no reason to) can increase the risk of a child developing a food allergy. It is better for the gastrointestinal tract (gut) of a baby and young child to be exposed to a variety of food allergens through a diverse and healthy diet.

Real Life Parenting

At 9 months old, Dina's daughter was found sneaking a lick of her stroller wheels (yikes!). Although Dina was dismayed, her daughter never got sick and Dina reminded herself that getting messy and exploring is how babies learn at this age. It's also possible that a young baby's exposure to germs may help strengthen the immune system.

...Y ALLERGENIC FOOD	FORM OF FOOD	SUGGESTED TIMING OF INTRODUCTION	OUR RECOMMENDATIONS
Milk *(These forms of milk apply only to exclusively breastfed infants as many formula-fed infants will drink milk-based formula.)*	Whole milk yogurt, no salt added ricotta, and cottage cheese	Before 1 year	6 months, after introduction of a few other foods
	Pieces of pasteurized cheese		8–12 months, or when eating finger foods
Soy	Pureed tofu or edamame	No special indication for delay	6–8 months
	Mashed tofu or edamame		8–12 months, or when eating finger foods
Wheat	Infant cereal	Before or by 6 months	6 months
Eggs	Pureed eggs	4–10 months	6–8 months
	Scrambled eggs, mashed hard-boiled eggs, eggs in baked goods		8–12 months, or when eating finger foods
Peanuts* *(in nut butter or dissolvable snack form; whole peanuts are potential choking hazards for infants)*	Peanut butter mixed with purees or in yogurt	6–12 months *Considerations are different for children who have a higher risk of peanut allergy	6–8 months, after introduction of a few other foods.
	Thin layer of peanut butter on crackers or dissolvable cereal snacks that contain peanut		8–12 months, or when eating finger foods
Tree nuts *(in nut butter or dissolvable snack form; whole nuts are potential choking hazards for infants)*	Nut butter mixed with purees or in yogurt	No special indication for delay	7–9 months, after introduction of other allergenic foods
	Thin layer of nut butter on a cracker or foods made with nut ingredients		9–12 months, or when eating finger foods
Fish	Pureed low-mercury fish (flaky white fish or salmon)	6–9 months	6–8 months
	Bite-sized pieces of boneless low-mercury fish		8–12 months, or when eating finger foods
Shellfish	Pureed low-mercury shellfish	No special indication for delay	6–8 months
	Crab cakes Soft bite-sized pieces of low-mercury shellfish		8–12 months, or when eating finger foods

Important Points About the Table on Page 86:

- It may not apply to infants who have any diagnosis of food allergies or other allergic diseases, or if there is a strong family history of allergies in the family. In these cases, you must discuss the introduction of allergenic foods with your pediatrician or allergist first, as allergy testing may be required prior to food introduction.
- There are no current published guidelines, so recommendations and suggested timing of introduction are based on current research and may change as more and better studies are published. An exception is peanut introduction.
- Allergenic foods should not be the first complementary foods added to a baby's diet. However, once your baby has started solids, if there is no reason to suspect your baby is at risk for food allergies, then you do not need to avoid allergenic foods.
- The initial small taste of an allergenic food should be given to a baby at home with a parent and not at a restaurant or park where medications are not readily available. If there is no sign of allergy, the portion size can be increased gradually with each subsequent feeding.

Allergists currently suggest that for a child who is *not* at any increased allergic risk, allergenic foods can be introduced at any time, in any order, in a matter that is appropriate for a child's age.

However, with all this said, we personally have practical recommendations for when these foods should be introduced (see "Introduction of the Highly Allergenic Foods" on page 86). Although the research reports you may introduce foods in any order, many physicians are still conservative and have their own opinions on when to give babies certain foods (medicine is often an art as well as a science).

Is there a time that I should introduce wheat to prevent celiac disease?

As with other allergenic foods, there is no evidence to suggest that delaying introduction of wheat beyond 6 months prevents food allergies or other allergic conditions. Current data does not show any difference in the prevalence of celiac disease in children who were given gluten at 6 months versus at 12 months of life. Therefore, we recommend introduction of gluten containing grains including infant barley, wheat, and multigrain cereal at 6 months of life.

What is food protein–induced enterocolitis?

As your baby begins to eat solids, he/she may not tolerate a food for a variety of reasons. If your child experiences repetitive or persistent vomiting and diarrhea after eating a food, that is significant enough to lead to dehydration, your child may have a condition called food protein–induced enterocolitis (FPIES.)

FPIES usually begins upon introduction of solid foods (around 4 to 6 months of age) and typically involves repetitive vomiting and diarrhea that starts several hours after a child eats the causative food. Sometimes the symptoms may be confused with a stomach virus. Although children with FPIES often do not have a fever, occasionally they may appear ill enough to warrant a visit to the emergency room. The good news is that children usually outgrow FPIES by 3 to 5 years of age and, though the symptoms of vomiting and diarrhea can be severe, the reaction is not associated with anaphylaxis.

What is the treatment for FPIES? What foods need to be avoided?

The main treatment for FPIES is fluid hydration. The vomiting reaction will eventually stop on its own, while the diarrhea may persist for several more hours.

FPIES is most commonly triggered by rice, wheat, oat, sweet potato, and poultry, but can also happen in the first months of life when your baby drinks milk or soy formulas. Other fruits and vegetables may also cause a FPIES reaction. It is also not unusual for a FPIES reaction to occur upon trying a food for the third or fourth time. Generally, a child does not have more than one to three foods that trigger FPIES reactions. A child with a suspected FPIES reaction should be evaluated by an allergist or pediatric gastroenterologist familiar with this condition. At this point, we still have a lot to learn about FPIES and there is active research into this unusual form of food allergy.

Stooling Patterns

While your baby is only drinking breast milk or formula, his/her stool is often watery or very soft, and the consistency of peanut butter. With the introduction of complementary foods, many parents are surprised at how different a baby's bowel movements will now look (and smell!). This section discusses normal colors and consistency of stools when starting solids.

Gastroesophageal Reflux at this Age

We reviewed reflux in detail in chapter one (see page 43). GER usually peaks at 4 to 5 months, and by 4 to 6 months, spitting up and vomiting should begin to improve. If your child was born prematurely, it may take longer to resolve. However, there are a few reasons why reflux may get worse at this age, including diet and a history of infections. With the introduction of more foods, your child may be consuming foods that are higher in acid, which may increase reflux symptoms. Also, a cold, ear infection, or other illness may affect how your child's stomach empties and may lead to worsening reflux symptoms. If symptoms are severe, causing discomfort or decreased intake and weight loss, speak to your pediatrician about dietary and medical therapies. If your child is already on medications, medication doses may need to be adjusted during this time as well.

I started solid foods and my baby's stool has changed. Is this normal?

It is completely normal for your child's stool pattern to change when solid foods are added to the diet, and the consistency of stool may become thicker or harder. Iron-fortified cereals are often added to the diet first. Rice cereal can lead to firmer stool and potentially aggravate constipation, while oatmeal cereal can lead to more gas. Please see chapters one and six for more information on constipation.

My baby's poop is green. Should I be worried?

Stool can be green, yellow, or brown in color. Worrisome colors include gray, tan, clay, pale yellow, or white, which may be associated with liver issues, or black and red, which may indicate blood. With liver disease, your child's skin and whites of the eyes may also appear yellow in color. Black stool may be a sign of old blood, while red streaks in the stool are most commonly due to hard stool causing tears known as rectal fissures. When your baby's stool looks a different color, try to remember what your child has recently eaten or whether your baby is on any new medications, since some medications and food may affect stool color. Also, when your child is sick, stool color may change and may temporarily contain mucus. If your baby's poop has changed, always express your concerns to your pediatrician. Doctors may look at a dirty diaper brought in to the office, so that together you can determine the cause of the stool changes.

Possible Causes of Change in Stool Color

COLOR OF STOOL	POSSIBLE FOOD	POSSIBLE MEDICATIONS
Black*	Blackberries, blueberries	Iron supplements, bismuth
Red*	Beets, cranberries, rhubarb, tomatoes, watermelon	Amoxicillin, Cefdinir, Rifampin
Green	Formula (fortified with iron), spinach, and other green leafy veggies	Grape-flavored Pedialyte
White/Light gray*	None	Antacids such as aluminum hydroxide (Maalox, Gaviscon)

Remember that although black, red, and gray or white poop may be due to food or medications, these colors may also be a sign of sickness and should always be discussed with your pediatrician

Mucus in Stool

Mucus in the stool may be normal and occur for a variety of reasons. Increased saliva or secretion production, colds, or teething may all lead to mucousy stools. Stomach bugs, as well as food allergies, are other possible reasons. If the mucousy stools persist, take a picture of it or bring a dirty diaper to your pediatrician to discuss it further.

Healthy Recipes for 4 to 6 Months

Starting solids is a fun and messy experience! This section contains recipes for your beginner eater. As we have stated before, there is no right order to introduce new purees, but we recommend offering only one new food every three to five days so if your child has a reaction, you can better identify the food that may have caused it. In addition, since some parents may have a small baby and a toddler to feed, each recipe in this section can be used as a double duty, so you can transform your baby's puree into a meal or a snack for your older child (or you!). Each of the recipes also has helpful nutrition facts. Although there are no standard recommendations for fiber intake for this age group, we will note when certain recipes contain fiber to help regulate your child's bowel habits.

To increase fiber content in the recipes, we kept skins on fruits and vegetables whenever feasible.

For these recipes, we make the claim that a recipe is a "good source" of a certain nutrient when the serving size we list meets ten to nineteen percent of the Dietary Reference Intake (DRI) for 4 to 6 month olds. We claim a recipe is an "excellent source" of a nutrient when the serving size listed meets twenty percent or more of the DRI for babies 4 to 6 month old. For double duty recipes, we will list the nutrition facts for toddlers 1 to 3 years old.

Using Breast Milk in Purees

The nutrition data for the recipes was calculated using water to thin the puree to the desired consistency. However, if you thin the puree with breast milk or formula, here is the approximate nutrition data for a tablespoon of breast milk or formula:

Calories: 10.8
Fat: 0.7 gram
Protein: 0.2 gram
Carbohydrate: 1 gram

Freezing Purees

We love to freeze purees in ice cube trays, which often hold 2 tablespoons of puree in each cube, the perfect serving size! After cleaning the ice cube tray well and letting the puree cool, you can place the puree in the ice cube tray and cover it with the ice cube tray cover or plastic wrap. Once frozen, you can move the cubes of food to labeled freezer bags and freeze for up to 1 month. Remember, defrosted food should not be refrozen.

Prune Puree

One of the first fruits we recommend is prunes. Constipation is a common issue that often arises in babies first starting solid foods. Since prunes are a good source of soluble and insoluble fiber, they have a laxative effect and are helpful in aiding normal bowel movements. If your baby develops constipation from other foods, prunes may be given to help regulate their stools. | MAKES 6 SERVINGS

12 pitted prunes, coarsely chopped

¾ cup water

Prep time: 5 minutes

Cook time: 5 minutes

Excellent source for 4- to 6-month-olds of iron, vitamin K, and potassium.

Check to make sure the prunes are truly pitted to avoid a choking hazard. Place the prunes and water in a saucepan and boil until the prunes are soft, approximately 5 minutes. Cool and blend the prunes until they are smooth and thin in consistency. Add more water to thin the puree if needed.

Refrigerate for up to 2 days or freeze for up to 1 month.

Note

We often also recommend roasting fruits and vegetables to bring out natural flavors prior to pureeing. See the butternut squash recipe (page 98) for cooking instructions although times and temperatures will vary. Here is list of good stage 1 purees:

Fruits: apple, apricot, avocado, banana, blueberry, pear, mango, and peach
Vegetables: corn, peas, and sweet potato
Meats: chicken, beef, lamb, pork, and turkey

We limited the serving size for this recipe to one tablespoon because each serving contains two prunes, which provides a sufficient amount of nutrients for this age group.

NUTRIENTS PER SERVING: 1 serving: 1 tablespoon • Calories: 45.6 • Total Fat: 0.1 g • Saturated Fat: 0 g • Protein: 0.4 g • Carbohydrates: 12.1 g • Sugar: 7.2 g • Vitamin K: 11.3 mcg • Fiber: 1.4 g • Iron: 0.2 mg • Sodium: 0.4 mg • Calcium: 8.2 mg • Potassium: 139.1 mg • **Provides 1 fruit serving per day for infants 4 to 6 months.**

Double Duty: Prune Pops

Prune ice pops are a delicious way to help your older infant and toddler when they have bouts of constipation. Pour 1 ounce (2 tablespoons) of the prune puree into each section of an ice cube tray. Freeze for one hour and then insert a lollipop stick into each cup so that the stick can stand up well on its own. Freeze for an additional five hours until puree is firm.

Real Life Parenting

Once Sebastian enjoyed oatmeal, Anthony added prune puree to the oatmeal and offered it to Sebastian for breakfast. This meal became one of Sebastian's favorites for the first year of his life. Now that he is eating table foods, he enjoys the puree as a dipping sauce for pancakes. Feel free to get creative with new combos of food as your child gets older.

NUTRIENTS PER SERVING FOR TODDLERS: 1 serving: 2 tablespoons • Calories: 91.2 • Total Fat: 0.2 g • Saturated Fat: 0 g • Protein: 0.8 g • Carbohydrates: 24.2 g • Sugar: 14.4 g • Vitamin K: 22.6 mcg • Fiber: 2.8 g • Iron: 0.4 mg • Sodium: 0.8 mg • Calcium: 16.4 mg • Potassium: 278.2 mg • **Provides ½ fruit serving per day for children 12 months to three years old.**

Mango Apricot Puree

After your baby has had no reaction to a few single ingredient purees, it is time to start experimenting with multiple ingredient purees. Have fun trying new combinations based on your child's taste preferences. Fresh fruit, such as mangos and apricots, make a perfect combination for their natural sweetness and fiber and are great first fruits for you baby to enjoy. | MAKES ABOUT ¾ CUP

1 cup fresh mango (about 1), peeled and cubed

½ cup fresh apricot (about 2) or may substitute peach (about ½), cubed

¼ cup water

Preheat oven to 400°F. Line a baking sheet with parchment paper. Place the fruit on the parchment paper and roast for 15 minutes or until they become soft. Let cool. Using a blender or immersion blender, process the fruit, including all of its juice from the pan. Add ¼ cup or more water to the puree, if needed, to reach desired consistency.

Refrigerate for up to two days and freeze for up to one month.

Prep time: 5 minutes

Cook time: 15 minutes

Excellent source for 4- to 6-month-olds of vitamin C, vitamin K, and iron.

Good source for 4- to 6-month-olds of folate and potassium.

NUTRIENTS PER SERVING: 1 serving: 2 tablespoons • Calories: 22.1 • Total Fat: 0.2 g • Saturated Fat: 0 g • Protein: 0.4 g • Carbohydrates: 5.4 g • Sugar: 4.8 g • Vitamin C: 11.2 mg • Folate: 12.9 mcg • Vitamin K: 1.5 mcg • Fiber: 0.7 g • Iron: 0.1 mg • Sodium: 0.4 mg • Calcium: 4.5 mg • Potassium: 76.4 mg • **Provides 1 fruit serving for infants 4 to 6 months.**

Double Duty: Mango Apricot Yogurt Parfait

We love using extra puree as a topping or dipping sauce for toddlers and adults alike (think dipping sauce for pancakes instead of syrup or a topping for oatmeal). We do not want any yummy drop of extra puree to go to waste! Here we use the mango apricot puree to make a delicious yogurt parfait for you and your toddlers. For adults, you can use regular granola without grinding it. | MAKES 1 SERVING

In a bowl or glass, layer the yogurt and puree and top with granola.

½ cup plain whole milk yogurt (may substitute vanilla yogurt)

¼ cup Mango Apricot Puree

2 tablespoons granola, finely ground (may substitute crushed Cheerios for younger toddlers)

Prep time: 2 minutes

NUTRIENTS PER SERVING FOR TODDLERS: 1 serving: 1 parfait • Calories: 193.2 • Total Fat: 8 g • Saturated Fat: 3.2 g • Protein: 7.3 g • Carbohydrates: 24.6 g • Sugar: 18.2 g • Vitamin C: 23 mg • Folate: 46.6 mcg • Vitamin K: 4.6 mcg • Fiber: 2.7 g • Iron: 0.9 mg • Sodium: 60.9 mg • Calcium: 169.2 mg • Potassium: 424.4 mg • **Provides** ½ dairy serving, ½ fruit serving, and ⅛ carbohydrate serving for children ages 1 to 3 years.

P2 Puree

Peaches and pears are high in fiber and are great to give if your child is constipated. We also like mixing the puree with iron-fortified oatmeal or barley cereal instead of rice cereal, which can be more binding. Always make sure to check the cereal ingredients if your child has food allergies, since some infant cereals may contain soy. | MAKES 1 TO 1½ CUPS

2 medium peaches, skin on, pitted and quartered

2 medium pears, skin on, seeded and quartered

Water

1 tablespoon iron-fortified oatmeal cereal

4-5 tablespoons of breast milk or formula

Prep time: 10 minutes

Cook time: 20 minutes

Excellent source for 4- to 6-month-olds of iron.

Good source for 4- to 6-month-olds of potassium.

Preheat the oven to 400°F.

Spread the fruit out on a parchment-line baking sheet. Roast the fruit for 20 minutes. Cool and puree the roasted fruit and add water to achieve desired consistency.

In a separate bowl, add 1 tablespoon of the cereal and mix it with 4 to 5 tablespoons of formula, water, or expressed breast milk until the cereal is thin and soup-like. Add 1 tablespoon of the puree to the prepared cereal and mix.

Refrigerate the puree without the cereal for up to 2 days, or freeze for up to 1 month. If milk was added to final mixture, may refrigerate for 24 hours.

Note

Like the prune puree, the P2 puree can also be frozen and made into ice pops for your older infant and toddler. Pour 1 ounce (2 tablespoons) of the puree into a cup of an ice cube tray. Freeze for one hour and then insert a lollipop stick into each cup so that the stick can stand up well on its own. Freeze for an additional five hours, until puree is firm. Each ice pop provides approximately half of a fruit serving per day for children one to three years old.

NUTRIENTS PER SERVING: 1 serving: 1 tablespoon fruit puree and 1 tablespoon prepared cereal (with formula or breast milk added) • Calories: 27.5 • Total Fat: 0.7 g • Saturated Fat: 0.3 g • Protein: 0.4 g • Carbohydrates: 5.5 g • Sugar: 4 g • Fiber: 0.8 g • Iron: 0.1 mg • Sodium: 2.1 mg • Calcium: 12.8 mg • Potassium: 48.4 mg • **Provides 1 fruit serving and 1 carbohydrate serving for infants 4 to 6 months.**

Double Duty: P2 Smoothie

We love doubling the P2 puree and freezing it for later use. Blended with a frozen banana and milk, it makes a delicious smoothie for breakfast or a snack.

| MAKES 4 CUPS

Blend the frozen P2 puree and frozen banana together and gradually add in milk. Blend until there are no more pieces of frozen fruit and mixture is smooth and creamy, 3 to 5 minutes.

Freeze in a covered container for up to 1 month.

½ to 1 cup P2 Puree, frozen

1 banana, chopped, frozen

1 cup whole milk

Prep time: 5 minutes

NUTRIENTS PER SERVING FOR TODDLERS: 1 serving: ½ cup • Calories: 46.7 • Total Fat: 1.1 g • Saturated Fat: 0.6 g • Protein: 1.3 g • Carbohydrates: 8.7 g • Sugar: 6 g • Fiber: 1.1 g • Iron: 0.1 mg • Sodium: 13.3 mg • Calcium: 37.1 mg • Potassium: 132.4 mg • Provides ¼ fruit serving and ⅛ dairy serving for children 1 to 3 years.

Roasted Butternut Squash Puree

Butternut squash is sweet and has a low risk of allergy. However, since it is a high-nitrate food, we recommend waiting until your child is 6 months of age before making it. It is a good source of fiber for your infant, which is useful for maintaining regular soft stools. We love precut butternut squash for this recipe; it is a big timesaver. | MAKES ABOUT 2½ CUPS

1 medium butternut squash, halved, or 32 ounces pre-cut and cubed butternut squash

¼ cup water, plus more for thinning

Prep time: 10 minutes

Cook time: 30 to 40 minutes

Excellent source for 4- to 6-month-olds of vitamin A, potassium, and iron.

Good source for 4- to 6-month-olds of vitamins C, E, and K, and folate.

Preheat the oven to 400°F.

If using whole squash, lay the butternut squash halves face down in a baking dish lined with parchment paper. Bake for 35 to 40 minutes. When the skin looks darker in color and the squash is soft enough to slide a knife in and out, remove from the oven. When the squash is cool enough to touch, scoop out the seeds and discard them. Then scoop out the flesh from the skin, placing it aside to cool. Discard the skin.

If using precut squash, spread the squash on a parchment-lined baking sheet and bake for 30 to 40 minutes, or until the squash becomes soft enough to slide a knife in and out. Set aside and let cool.

After the flesh has cooled, using a food processor, regular blender, or immersion blender, begin to puree. Add ¼ cup of water or more to achieve desired texture.

Refrigerate for up to 1 day or freeze for up to 1 month.

NUTRIENTS PER SERVING: 1 serving: 2 tablespoons • Calories: 14.2 • Total Fat: 0 g • Saturated Fat: 0 g • Protein: 0.3 g • Carbohydrates: 3.7 g • Sugar: 0.7 g • Vitamin A: 167.4 mcg • Vitamin C: 6.6 mg • Vitamin E: 0.5 mg • Vitamin K: 0.4 mg • Folate: 8.5 mcg • Iron: 0.2 mg • Fiber: 0.6 g • Sodium: 1.3 mg • Potassium: 110.9 mg • Calcium: 15.1 mg • **Provides 1 vegetable serving for 6-month-old infants.**

Double Duty: Spiced Butternut Squash Soup

You can roast extra butternut squash to make a soup for the rest of the family. This provides a hearty meal with little extra effort. This recipe is for parents and toddlers but can easily be adjusted to give to your baby—just leave out the honey and the salt! | MAKES ABOUT 10 CUPS

Heat the oil in a large pot on medium-high heat. Sauté the onion, carrots, and apples until the onions become translucent, about 5 minutes. Add the water, salt, cinnamon, curry, vanilla, and honey. Bring to a boil and then lower to a simmer, cooking for 15 minutes until the apples and carrots have softened. Add the butternut squash puree and let simmer an additional 5 minutes until all the flavors are combined. Remove from the heat, cool, and puree the soup in batches using an immersion or regular blender until smooth. Serve warm.

Refrigerate for up to 3 days or freeze for up to 3 months.

2 tablespoons olive oil

1 medium yellow onion, diced

1½ medium carrots, peeled and diced (about 1 cup)

5 medium Gala apples, peeled, cored, and diced (about 4 cups)

5 cups water

1¾ teaspoons salt

½ teaspoon ground cinnamon

¼ teaspoon mild curry powder

1 teaspoon vanilla extract

¼ cup honey

2 cups butternut squash puree

Prep time: 10 minutes

Cook time: 25 minutes

NUTRIENTS PER SERVING FOR TODDLERS: 1 serving: ¾ cup • Calories: 91.6 • Total Fat: 2.3 g • Saturated Fat: 0.3 g • Protein: 0.7 g • Carbohydrates: 18.9 g • Sugar: 12.9 g • Vitamin A: 260.1 mcg • Vitamin C: 11.4 mg • Vitamin E: 0.9 mg • Vitamin K: 1.8 mg • Folate: 13.3 mcg • Iron: 0.4 mg • Fiber: 2 g • Sodium: 317.4 mg • Potassium: 226.7 mg • Calcium: 27 mg • Provides ½ vegetable serving and ½ fruit serving for children ages 1 to 3 years.

Zucarrot Puree

Once your child has tried zucchini and carrots separately, you can start mixing them together into a new tasty flavor combination. Carrots are a great source of vitamin A, zucchini provides vitamin C, and both provide fiber for your infant. As carrots may contain nitrates, we recommend this puree at around 6 months. | MAKES 1½ TO 2 CUPS

2 zucchinis, chopped (approximately 2 cups)

5 carrots, peeled and chopped (approximately 2 cups)

Water

Prep time: 10 minutes

Cook time: 40 to 50 minutes

Excellent source for 4- to 6-month-olds of vitamins A and K, iron, and potassium.

Good source for 4- to 6-month-olds of vitamin C and folate.

Preheat the oven to 400°F.

Spread the zucchini and carrots on two separate parchment-lined baking sheets. Roast the carrots for 40 to 50 minutes, or until soft, and roast the zucchini for 25 to 30 minutes, until soft. Cool and blend until the mixture is smooth and has a thin consistency. Add water to thin the puree.

Refrigerate for up to 1 day or freeze for up to 1 month.

NUTRIENTS PER SERVING: 1 serving: 2 tablespoons • Calories: 13.7 • Total Fat: 0.1 g • Saturated Fat: 0 g • Protein: 0.5 g • Carbohydrates: 3 g • Sugar: 1.7 g • Vitamin A: 184.8 mcg • Vitamin C: 6.3 mg • Vitamin K: 4.1 mcg • Folate: 10.9 mcg • Iron: 0.2 mg • Fiber: 0.9 g • Sodium: 17.3 mg • Calcium: 11.7 mg • Potassium: 142.8 mg • Provides 1 vegetable serving for 6-month-old infants.

Double Duty: Zucarrot Soufflé

Turn your zucarrot puree into a healthy side-dish for older babies, toddlers, and adults! This tasty combination is a good way to get your toddler to eat veggies and fiber! | MAKES 6 SERVINGS

Preheat the oven to 350°F.

Line an 8-inch square pan with parchment paper. Heat the oil in a small saucepan and sauté the onions on medium heat until they begin to turn brown. In a bowl, mix together the egg and cheese. Add the flour and salt. Combine the puree with the cheese mixture. Add the onions and mix well. Pour into the prepared pan and bake for about 1 hour, or until the top is browned and crusted.

Refrigerate for up to 3 days or freeze for up to 1 month.

1 tablespoon olive oil

¼ small onion, minced

1 egg, whisked

4 oz mozzarella cheese, shredded, full fat

1 tablespoon whole-wheat or all-purpose flour

¼ teaspoon salt (for toddlers and adults)

1½ to 2 cups of Zucarrot Puree

Prep time: 10 minutes

Cook time: 70 minutes

NUTRIENTS PER SERVING: 1 serving: 4 by 2.5-inch square • Calories: 98.3 • Total Fat: 5.6 g • Saturated Fat: 1.9 g • Protein: 4.6 g • Carbohydrates: 8.3 g • Sugar: 4.1 g • Vitamin A: 461.2 mcg • Vitamin C: 14.9 mg • Vitamin K: 9.8 mcg • Folate: 31 mcg • Fiber: 2.2 g • Iron: 0.6 mg • Sodium: 209.1 mg • Calcium: 80.1 mg • Potassium: 360.6 mg • Provides ¼ protein serving, ⅔ dairy serving, and ¾ vegetable serving for children 1 to 3 years.

Roasted Banana and Greek Yogurt Puree

At around 6 months and after your baby has eaten several fruits and vegetables, yogurt is a great protein to introduce. We recommend giving plain baby or whole milk yogurt or whole Greek yogurt and adding your own pureed fruit or vegetable to it (store-bought flavored baby yogurt often has unnecessary added sugar). Greek yogurt can often be a bit tart, so we like mixing it with sweet bananas for a quick and easy lunch and added potassium and iron to the diet. Roasting the banana brings out a richer flavor.

Bananas can also be helpful if your child has loose stools. If your baby tends to be constipated, however, we recommend adding the yogurt to one of the "P" fruits instead, for example, prunes, pears, plums, or peaches. | MAKES ⅓ CUP

1 ripe banana, peeled and cut into ¼-inch slices

1 tablespoon full-fat Greek yogurt

Water

Prep time: 5 minutes

Cook time: 25 minutes

Excellent source for 4- to 6-month-olds of vitamin B₁₂, iron, and potassium.

Good source for 4- to 6-month-olds of protein.

For unroasted banana puree, blend the banana until smooth. Add 1 tablespoon of the puree to 1 tablespoon of Greek yogurt in a separate bowl. Add water, until it reaches the desired consistency.

For roasted banana puree, preheat the oven to 400°F. Arrange the banana slices in a single layer on a baking sheet lined with parchment paper. Bake until golden brown around the edges and soft in the middle, approximately 25 minutes. Once cooled, puree with an immersion or regular blender. Add 1 tablespoon of puree to 1 tablespoon of yogurt. Add water until it reaches the desired consistency.

The puree without the yogurt can be refrigerated for up to 2 days or frozen for up to 1 month.

Note

The roasted slices of banana, by themselves or with a thin smear of peanut butter, also make a great portable snack for toddlers!

NUTRIENTS PER SERVING: 1 serving: 1 tablespoon banana puree plus 1 tablespoon Greek yogurt • Calories: 38.6 • Total Fat: 1.5 g • Saturated Fat: 1.2 g • Protein: 1.2 g • Carbohydrates: 5.5 g • Sugar: 3.2 g • Vitamin B₁₂: 0.1 mcg • Fiber: 0.6 g • Iron: 0.1 mg • Sodium: 4.3 mg • Calcium: 13.6 mg • Potassium: 79.7 mg • **Provides 1 fruit serving and 1 protein serving for 6-month-old infants.**

Double Duty: Banana Bites

We loved fruit roll-ups in our lunch boxes as a child, but as parents now we don't like all the added sugars and extra ingredients in snacks. This easy recipe, reminiscent of a roll-up but in bite-sized pieces for young children, results in a fun finger food that can be enjoyed by the whole family! | MAKES 5 SERVINGS

Preheat the oven to 225°F.

Spread the pureed bananas about ⅛ of an inch thin on a parchment-lined cookie sheet. Sprinkle with a pinch of cinnamon. Bake in the oven for a 1 to 1½ hours, until crispy. Let cool and break into bite-size pieces.

Store covered in airtight container in the refrigerator for up to 3 days.

2 bananas, pureed

Cinnamon

Prep time: 5 minutes

Cook time: 1 to 1½ hours

NUTRIENTS PER SERVING FOR TODDLERS: 1 serving: ⅕ of recipe • Calories: 42.2 • Total Fat: 0.2 g • Saturated Fat: 0.1 g • Protein: 0.5 g • Carbohydrates: 10.8 g • Sugar: 5.8 g • Fiber: 1.3 g • Sodium: 0.5 mg • Calcium: 3.1 mg • Potassium: 169.3 mg • Iron: 0.1 mg • **Provides ⅓ fruit serving per day for children ages 1 to 3 years.**

Chapter Three

7 to 8 Months

In chapter three, we will discuss your 7- to 8-month-old baby. As your child continues to increase his/her intake of solid foods, we will address common questions such as balancing solid food and milk intake, food refusal, introduction of spices, teething, what to do if your child is having difficulty gaining weight, and celiac disease. In this chapter, we also give a typical menu for this age group and recipes for more experienced eaters with expanding textures and flavors.

Expected Developmental Milestones

Your baby will be developing by leaps and bounds now! Motor strength increases and your child will love to stand on his/her legs and bounce up and down on your lap. Your baby is rolling over both ways, tripoding (using his/her arms to help sit up) like a champ, and will soon sit all on his/her own. Around this time, your baby will develop full color vision and will see long distances away. Socially, your baby will love to explore and put everything in his/her mouth, will enjoy watching him/herself in the mirror, respond to your emotions by your tone of voice, and be joyful most of the time. Cognitively, your baby will begin to understand more and may respond to his/her own name, will babble, and imitate sounds.

Developmental Milestones for 7–8 Months

AGE	MOTOR AND VISUAL SKILLS	SOCIAL SKILLS	COGNITIVE/ LANGUAGE
7–8 months	Stands on legs and bounces up and down on caregiver's lap, may start to sit up on own. Develops full color vision, sees long distances away, and eyesight nearly mature.	Loves to explore and put everything in his/her mouth, enjoys watching him/herself in the mirror, responds to caregiver's emotions by tone of voice, and is joyful most of the time.	May respond to his/her own name, babbles, and imitates sounds.

FEEDING SKILLS

Easily eats from spoon and able to eat thicker textures, attempts to grasp foods and transfer food from hand to hand, may control where food is located in mouth, drinks messily from cup.

Basic Nutritional Guidelines

Your little one is loving his/her first foods and is quickly becoming a pro at eating simple purees. We discuss in this section how to balance complementary foods with breast milk or formula intake, what your baby should be eating at this stage, and how to introduce spices.

Typical Menu for 7 to 8 Months

This menu is an example of what your child's intake may be at this age, but may vary based on your child's developmental readiness for new foods.

Range of Calories per Day	
AGE	CALORIES PER DAY*
7–8 Months	Males: 668–746
	Females: 608–678

This range of calories is an estimate based on the average child. Your child may require more or less calories.

Adapted from USDA Food and Nutrition Service's Infant Nutrition and Feeding Guide for Use in the WIC and CSF Programs.

Early Morning: Breastfeeding or 6 to 8 ounces breast milk or formula

Breakfast: 1 to 2 tablespoons of cereal plus 1 to 2 tablespoons stage 1 or 2 fruit

Mid-morning: Breastfeeding or 6 to 8 ounces breast milk or formula

Lunch: Breastfeeding or 6 to 8 ounces breast milk or formula

Late afternoon: Breastfeeding or 6 to 8 ounces breast milk or formula

Dinner: 1 to 2 tablespoons of cereal plus 1 to 2 tablespoons stage 1 or 2 vegetables, fruit or protein

Bedtime: Breastfeeding or 6 to 8 ounces breast milk or formula

Totals:

Milk intake: 3 to 5 feeds; approximately 24 to 32 ounces per day

Grains: 2 to 3 servings (1 serving: 1 to 2 tablespoons).

Fruits and vegetables: 1 to 2 servings (1 serving: 1 to 2 tablespoons).

Proteins: 1 serving (1 serving: 1 to 2 tablespoons).

Balancing Solid Foods with Breast Milk or Formula

Generally, babies will drink six to eight ounces or will breastfeed three to five times a day at this age and will gradually decrease their milk intake as their consumption of solid food increases. Most babies will breastfeed or have formula when they wake up, followed by breakfast thirty to forty-five minutes later. Some babies, however, may prefer to eat breakfast first, followed by breast milk or formula. More milk is offered prior to lunch, followed by lunch (which may consist of either breast milk or formula or additional solid food), milk after a nap, solid food for dinner, and the last breastfeeding or formula prior to bedtime. This is just a guideline—we always suggest going by your baby's cues and coming up with a nutrition plan with the help of your pediatrician.

What should my baby be eating now?

Now that your baby is getting the hang of eating solid foods, the food can be thicker and less soupy in consistency with a chunkier texture. More combinations of foods can be introduced, as long as your baby has not had an allergic reaction to the individual components. At this age your child should be eating a variety of foods from all major food groups.

When can I start giving my baby spices?

If you have been breastfeeding, your baby has already been exposed to the spices you have been eating and has been "tasting" them through your breast milk. It is definitely okay to add spices to solid foods and there is no reason a baby should be only eating a bland diet. We still recommend the old rule of trying one new food or spice every three to five days, so that you can easily identify the culprit if an allergy develops. Spices are a rare allergy, but they do occur and can be severe, just like any food allergy. Mustard allergy, for example, may be more common in children who have sesame or other seed allergies. If your child is allergic to any seeds, make sure to check the list of ingredients and spices carefully, since they do not fall under the labeling of the Food Allergen Labeling and Consumer Protection Act (see sidebar, page 109).

Some common spices and herbs to start with are cinnamon, nutmeg, vanilla (from the bean or from an extract if flavoring the food, since pure vanilla may contain alcohol, but if the food is cooked after adding vanilla, the alcohol will usually evaporate), allspice, mint, garlic, oregano, basil, parsley, rosemary, cilantro, dill, and thyme. After trying a few of the gentler spices, if you normally cook with the "spicier" spices, you could even try options like curry powder, coriander, ginger, and chile, or anything that you normally cook with for your family's meals. The only seasonings we would stay away from are salt and sugar, which we will discuss in chapter five.

Allergens on Food Labels

The Food Allergen Labeling and Consumer Protection Act (FALCPA) states that food labels must clearly list major food allergens (milk, eggs, fish, shellfish, peanuts, tree nuts, wheat, and soybeans) in the ingredient list, by using the word "contains" before the allergen, or by having the common allergen in parentheses by the name of the food from which it is derived in the list of ingredients, such as "albumin (egg)." Certain raw agricultural commodities including fresh fruit and vegetables and refined oils may be exempt from this provision.

What do I do if my child refuses a food?

Many babies will grimace when trying a new food for the first time. Don't despair! It may take ten or even twenty tries before your baby likes the new food. Sometimes it is helpful to add a bit of an old favorite with a soon-to-be new favorite. For instance, mixing some new pureed chicken with his/her beloved applesauce may be a hit, or adding a dash of cinnamon, which you know your baby already likes, to Greek yogurt may do the trick. If your baby still refuses the food, wait a few days and try again.

My baby's skin looks orange, is something wrong?

If your baby's skin has an orange tinge, usually seen on the nose, palms, and soles, it could be a benign condition called carotenemia caused by your baby's diet. It is due to eating high amounts of healthy beta-carotene-rich foods like carrots, sweet potatoes, pumpkin, and squash and is usually not a cause of concern. The orange discoloration will resolve within weeks of diet changes. Although these foods are rich in vitamin A, vitamin A toxicity would be rare. Even though carotenemia is relatively common, we still recommend that your pediatrician look at your infant's skin further to make sure your baby isn't jaundiced or has a very rare, more serious alternate cause of carotenemia.

Teething

Most babies will develop teeth between 4 and 12 months, but there is a wide variation of when a first tooth may appear and some babies may have no teeth by their first birthday. The following questions discusses how to comfort your child when they are teething and when to start brushing your child's teeth.

My baby seems to be teething. Can I give him/her a teething biscuit? How else can I make my baby feel better?

You may offer a teething biscuit, but keep in mind it is not very nutritious and you have to watch your baby while he/she is eating the biscuit, since chunks may break off easily. Also, most brands have sugar and salt (yes, even the organic ones) and why start off right away exposing your baby's first shiny tooth to sugar? For example, one popular teething cracker contains organic rice flour, sugar, and salt and does not report containing any vitamins or minerals. Alternatively, you can massage your child's gums with clean fingers or offer teething rings or a clean frozen or wet washrag. Discuss with your pediatrician if acetaminophen (Tylenol) might be appropriate on those really rough days. We recommend staying away from teething tablets that contain the plant poison belladonna and gels with benzocaine. Belladonna and benzocaine are marketed to numb your child's pain, but the FDA has issued warnings against both due to potential side effects. We, as well as the American Academy of Pediatrics (AAP), do not recommend amber teething necklaces since we don't suggest placing any product around an infant's neck that can pose a strangulation risk or be a potential choking hazard, especially since there is no research backing the necklace's effectiveness.

How often should I brush my child's teeth?

Once your child develops teeth, you should be brushing them twice a day with a smear of fluoride toothpaste the size of a grain of rice, especially after the last drink of the day. In most cases, you should also make your first dental appointment when the first tooth erupts or by a year of age (the AAP and the American Academy of Pediatric Dentistry recommends a "dental home" by 1 year old, though some dentists may recommend to wait until 3 years of life). After 3 years of age, it is recommended to use a pea-size amount of fluoride toothpaste when brushing.

Expected Growth

Your child's weight gain will continue to slow down after 6 months of age and at 7 to 8 months your baby's normal rate of growth is not as rapid as when he/she was a few months old. In this section, we discuss what is appropriate growth and how to know if your child is growing well.

How much should my child be gaining at this age?

Between 6 and 12 months of age, your child will gain an average of 10 grams per day or 1 ounce every three days. Your child should gain approximately 1 pound every six weeks instead of the 1 pound per month that is expected between 3 to 6 months of age. Length will also increase at a slower rate, approximately $^3/_8$ inch per month, while head circumference will increase by approximately a $^1/_4$ centimeter per month until they are about 1 year old.

How do I know if my child is growing well for his age?

The most important way to determine if your child is eating enough or gaining enough weight is by reviewing his/her growth chart with the pediatrician. Pediatricians will often advise parents that it is normal for some children to be on the 10th percentile for weight while other children are on the 90th percentile. It is more important that your child follows his own curve and, more or less, grows along consistent percentiles. The World Health Organization (WHO) growth charts (pages 222–223) are now recommended for both formula fed and breastfed infants from birth until 2 years old.

Medical Concerns

Now that your child is on a more varied diet, many parents have concerns about whether their child is eating enough and gaining weight appropriately. This section discusses reasons why your child may not be gaining adequate weight for his/her age (a term known as *failure to thrive*) as well as providing examples of high calorie foods to incorporate into his/her diet. Also, now that children are eating gluten-containing (wheat, rye, barley) foods, parents often ask, "What are the signs to look out for in the development of celiac disease?" In this section, we will define celiac disease and explain how it differs from wheat allergy and gluten sensitivity. Finally, we end with a discussion on gastroesophageal reflux disease (GERD) and how to wean your child off of any medications for this condition, as GERD will likely be improving at this age.

Failure to Thrive

Your pediatrician may use the term *failure to thrive* (or FTT) to describe a child that is not gaining weight as expected for his or her age. Although this term may be scary for a parent to hear, there are many reasons why a child may not be gaining weight adequately, so do not be alarmed if your pediatrician labels your baby *failure to thrive*. FTT is just a term to identify those babies who need further evaluation to figure out why they are growing slowly and a plan to help them improve. Typically, FTT is defined as a child whose weight has crossed two major percentiles. Major percentiles are indicated by lines on growth charts and typically include the 3rd, 5th, 10th, 25th, 50th, 75th, and 95th percentiles. If your child was growing at the 75th percentile and dropped to the 25th percentile for weight, they would have crossed two major percentiles (from 75th to 50th to the 25th percentile) and may be considered *failure to thrive* (see chart, opposite).

What are the causes of failure to thrive?

The causes of FTT include insufficient caloric intake, increased caloric losses, and increased caloric need. The most common cause is due to behavioral issues around food, which may lead to insufficient caloric intake. Food allergies may also present with poor weight gain and insufficient caloric intake since these children may have difficulty ingesting enough calories if they are on such a limited diet. Children with chronic vomiting and/or diarrhea, such as in children with celiac disease, are examples of children who may have increased caloric losses. Although a less common cause of FTT, children who may have an increased caloric need include those with heart and kidney disease.

What is the treatment of failure to thrive?

We generally recommend a 24-hour diet recall or a 3-day calorie count done by either a dietitian or your pediatrician to assess if your child is getting enough calories. Other tests may be done to evaluate medical reasons for poor weight gain. Specific tests will vary depending on your child's age, past medical and family history, and if any other symptoms are present. In general, your doctor may check for celiac disease (as long as your child has eaten gluten), and assess for anemia, liver, thyroid, and kidney disease by performing blood work. In addition, if your child has diarrhea, your doctor may check his/her stool for protein, fat, and sugar to determine whether your child is adequately absorbing food. A referral to a pediatric gastroenterologist also may be suggested, especially if a child is vomiting, has diarrhea, gags with feeds, or is uncomfortable when they eat or stool.

The treatment for FTT varies depending on the underlying cause, which may need to be addressed before your child is able to gain weight appropriately. Children with FTT require increased calories and meals should be fortified with high calorie foods. Working with a health care professional and dietitian is important to ensure that your child is getting adequate calories.

If my child is not gaining weight appropriately, what are examples of high-calorie foods I can add to his/her diet?

High-calorie foods that can be added to the diet include options such as avocado, whole milk dairy products, heavy cream, nut butter, and natural oils. Coconut oil tastes great and can be added to your child's milk or pureed foods. Each tablespoon of coconut oil has 117 calories! There are also many

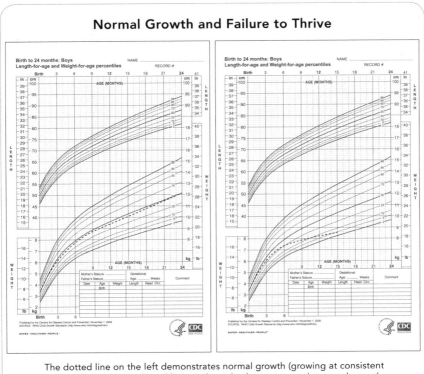

Normal Growth and Failure to Thrive

The dotted line on the left demonstrates normal growth (growing at consistent percentiles) while the dotted line on the right demonstrates decreased growth, where the weight percentile has decreased by two percentiles. Large versions of this chart appear on pages 222 and 223.

fortified nutritional supplements available in the form of milk and powdered supplements. Please see page 192 for specific examples. We recommend speaking with your pediatrician before using any of these products.

Celiac Disease

Celiac disease is a permanent gluten intolerance that can lead to inflammation in the small intestines. It is now more commonly being diagnosed in part because of improved awareness and screening tests. It is estimated to occur in 1 out of 133 people. Celiac disease can present as early as 6 to 8 months of life, after gluten has been introduced into the diet. It can present in the following ways:

- Gastrointestinal symptoms, which is the most common presentation for children from 6 to 24 months of life. Typical symptoms include vomiting, abdominal pain or bloating, poor weight gain, constipation, and diarrhea.
- Nongastrointestinal symptoms, including short stature (lower height than expected), rashes, and iron deficiency anemia that is not responsive to supplementation with iron therapy.
- Without any symptoms and is discovered on routine screening of certain children at increased risk of developing celiac disease, such as those with Trisomy 21/Down's syndrome, type 1 diabetes, and first-degree relatives (including parents and siblings) of those diagnosed with celiac disease.

How does celiac disease differ from wheat allergy?

Celiac disease is an immune-mediated disease where the presence of gluten causes an inflammatory response that irritates the lining of the small intestines. It is a lifelong condition and can be screened via reliable blood tests, along with a specific type of inflammation found on a biopsy of the small intestine.

Wheat allergy, on the other hand, is an IgE-mediated food allergy (along with milk, eggs, soy, peanuts, tree nuts, fish, and shellfish) and in some children can trigger immediate and possibly severe allergic reactions, including anaphylaxis (which is not seen in celiac disease). This type of allergy is diagnosed with different types of tests, including skin prick tests and a blood test to check specific IgE levels. Children with IgE-mediated wheat allergy must strictly avoid any exposure to wheat but in the majority of cases will be able to eat other gluten-containing grains.

What is gluten sensitivity?

Non-celiac gluten sensitivity lacks a clear definition. It is usually used for individuals who have symptoms following ingestion of gluten that resolve once gluten has been eliminated from the diet. Symptoms are similar to those seen in celiac disease. Common gastrointestinal complaints include gas, diarrhea, and constipation. Other symptoms seen in older children and adolescents include joint pain, headaches, rashes, and fatigue. The diagnosis should be made only after a consultation with your physician who will make sure your child does not have celiac disease or a wheat allergy.

The prevalence of non-celiac gluten sensitivity is not well known. In fact, some physicians question whether it is even a true entity. Some studies estimate that it may occur in as much as 8 percent of the overall population, while others estimate that it is quite rare in children.

Gluten sensitivity cannot be detected by celiac screening, intestinal biopsies, or standard allergy tests. In fact, all of these tests will likely be normal in individuals with gluten sensitivity. Although some practitioners may offer various (costly) alternative tests to diagnose non-celiac gluten sensitivity, so far there are no proven or reliable tests to confirm this diagnosis. Currently, the diagnosis of gluten sensitivity is predominantly a clinical one and is based on observed resolution of gastrointestinal and other symptoms following the removal of gluten from the diet. Please see chapter six for more details.

Gastroesophageal Reflux (GER)

By 7 months, GER should improve in most children. We, therefore, will discuss why and how to wean medications your child may be on for gastroesophageal reflux in this section.

I think my child's gastroesophageal reflux is improving, can I stop medications?

By this age, your child will be eating more solid food and learning to sit up by him- or herself. These are important developmental milestones that will help decrease spit-up episodes and vomiting. The lower esophageal muscle, however, will not reach its full length until about two years of life, so occasional spit-up and vomiting is still possible. Most children will be in less pain if they do spit up. Overall, GER should be improving at this stage but spit-up can worsen temporarily when children have a viral illness. If your child is on medications for GERD, and symptoms have improved, this may be a good time to speak to your pediatrician about when to wean the medication. Your pediatrician will decide whether to stop the medication altogether or wean the medication more slowly over a few days or weeks. (For more information on gastroesophageal reflux, see page 194.)

Healthy Recipes for 7 to 8 Months

Your 7- to 8-month-old is now experienced in chewing and ready for thicker textures, flavor combinations, and spices. Since children may have trouble gaining weight at this age, we also include ways to increase calories in these recipes. Finally, as there are no recommended fiber requirements for this age, we will note which recipes contain high amounts of fiber.

For these recipes, we make the claim that a recipe is a "good source" of a certain nutrient when the serving size we list meets 10 to 19 percent of the Dietary Reference Intake (DRI) for a 7- to 8-month-old. We claim a recipe is an "excellent source" of a nutrient when the serving size listed meets 20 percent or more of the DRI for a 7- to 8-month-old.

Sweet and Green Puree

This naturally sweet vegetable and fruit puree is packed with fiber and vitamin
This recipe provides a delicious way for babies to eat their greens! | MAKES 3 CUPS

Place the spinach, peas, pineapple, and pears in a
blender. Add the water and blend until the puree reaches
desired consistency, adding more water if necessary.

Refrigerate for up to 1 day or freeze for up to 1 month.

Note

This recipe contains pineapple, an acidic fruit. Some babies
with sensitive skin may develop a non-allergic contact rash.
Feel free to remove pineapple from the recipe or substitute
with another fruit if a significant rash develops.

To add calories, add 1 tablespoon of heavy cream to each
serving to provide an additional 52 calories, 0.3 grams of
protein, and 5.5 grams of fat.

**1 cup packed fresh
spinach leaves**

**½ cup frozen peas,
thawed**

**½ of a medium pineapple,
cubed (1½ cups)
(see Note)**

**2 pears, peel on,
seeded and cubed**

**½ cup water, plus more
if necessary**

Prep time: 10 minutes

Excellent source for
7- to 8-month-olds of
vitamin K.

Good source for
7- to 8-month-olds of
vitamin C, potassium,
and folate.

Real Life Parenting

When Dina first tried out this recipe on her favorite picky critics, Julia
and Evie, they could not stop eating it! Julia would sneak into the fridge
for it and even asked, "Do we *really* have to save some for Anthony to
taste?" Dina quickly learned this baby puree could also serve as a green
drink for toddlers (or adults!) or as a healthy ice pop on warm days.

NUTRIENTS PER SERVING: 1 serving: 4 tablespoons puree • Calories: 32/64 • Total Fat: 0 g/0.1 g • Saturated Fat:
0 g/0 g • Protein: 0.7 g/1.5 g • Carbohydrates: 7.9 g/15.7 g • Fiber: 1.7 g/3.3 g • Sugar: 5.3 g/10.5 g • Vitamin C:
5.3 mg/10.7 mg • Vitamin K: 25.6 mcg/51.2 mcg • Calcium: 14.2 mg/28.5 mg • Folate: 14.5 mcg/29.1 mcg • Iron:
0.3 mg/0.7 mg • Potassium: 104.8 mg/209.5 mg • Sodium: 8.3 mg/16.6 mg • Provides approximately 2 fruit servings
and 1 vegetable serving for infants 7 to 8 months. Provides ½ fruit serving and ¼ vegetable serving for children
1 to 3 years.

Banana-Avocado Fruity Puree

This is one of our favorite recipes for babies since it combines fruit and dairy with healthy fats and fiber. We also love this recipe for how convenient it is on those hectic mornings when you want to serve a nutritious breakfast but have limited time. This puree makes a perfect start to the day for your baby.

| MAKES ABOUT 1¼ CUPS

¾ cup plain full-fat Greek yogurt

½ banana, peeled

½ avocado, pitted and peeled

½ cup mixed berries (such as strawberries or blueberries, see Note)

Water

Prep time: 5 minutes

Excellent source for 7- to 8-month-olds of protein and vitamins B₁₂ and K.

Good source for 7- to 8-month-olds of vitamin C and potassium.

Blend the yogurt, banana, avocado, and berries until smooth. Add water until it reaches desired consistency.

Refrigerate for up to 1 day (may cause some discoloration).

Note

Choose ripe fruit or fruits that you know your child loves since the sweetness of the recipe is dependent on the fruit.

To add calories, add 1 teaspoon of peanut butter to each serving to provide an additional 33 calories, 1.2 grams protein, and 2.7 grams fat.

NUTRIENTS PER SERVING: 1 serving: 3 tablespoons • Calories: 65.4 • Total Fat: 4.4 g • Saturated Fat: 2.2 g • Protein: 2.3 g • Carbohydrates: 5.2 g • Fiber: 1 g • Sugar: 2.6 g • Vitamin B₁₂: 0.1 mcg • Vitamin C: 5.3 mg • Vitamin K: 1.1 mcg • Calcium: 24.6 mg • Iron: 0.2 mg • Potassium: 98 mg • Sodium: 7.5 mg • **Provides approximately 1 fruit serving and 1 protein serving for infants 7 to 8 months.**

Blueberry-Pear Protein Puree

Quinoa (pronounced KEEN-wah) is often eaten like a grain, but it is actually a seed that is popular because it is nutrient dense and gluten-free. It is called a "complete protein" because it contains all the essential amino acids (the building blocks of protein). Quinoa can be incorporated into many recipes because of its subtle flavor, which can be easily manipulated by stronger flavors. Pears and blueberries add additional fiber, making this recipe a great combination puree with new textures and flavor blends. | MAKES 1½ CUPS

Preheat the oven to 400°F.

Spread the pears on a parchment-lined baking sheet and roast for 20 minutes, or until soft. Cool, then puree the pears and blueberries in a food processor or blender. Add water until the mixture reaches the desired consistency.

For each serving, add 4 tablespoons of puree to 4 teaspoons of cooked quinoa and blend, if needed.

Refrigerate for up to 2 days or freeze without quinoa for up to 1 month.

Note

To add calories, add 1 teaspoon of chia seeds to each serving to provide an additional 20 calories, 1.0 gram protein, and 1.5 grams fat.

2 pears, skin on, seeded, and cubed

1 cup blueberries

Water

½ cup cooked quinoa

Prep time: 5 minutes

Cook time: 20 minutes

Excellent source for 7- to 8-month-olds of vitamin K.

Good source for 7- to 8-month-olds of protein, folate, and potassium.

NUTRIENTS PER SERVING: 1 serving: 4 tablespoons fruit puree and 4 teaspoons quinoa • Calories: 65.9 • Total Fat: 0.4 g • Saturated Fat: 0 g • Protein: 1.2 g • Carbohydrates: 15.5 g • Fiber: 3 g • Sugar: 7.9 g • Vitamin K: 4.8 mcg • Calcium: 10.8 mg • Folate: 8 mcg • Iron: 0.3 mg • Sodium: 1.3 mg • **Provides approximately 1 carbohydrate serving and 2 fruit servings for infants 7 to 8 months.**

Dairy-Free Sweet Potato Pudding

Babies tend to love sweet potatoes and gravitate toward orange vegetables for their natural sweetness. We love them because they are not only tasty but also full of nutrition. The dates add to the sweetness and provide fiber, while the tofu is a good source of protein. | MAKES 1⅔ CUPS

2½ medium sweet potatoes

½ pound (½ a package) silken tofu, drained (make sure to only use silken)

¼ cup dates, pitted

1 teaspoon ground cinnamon

Water

Prep time: 5 minutes

Cook time: 45 to 60 minutes

Good source for 7- to 8-month-olds of protein, vitamin A, and potassium.

Preheat the oven to 400°F.

Prick each sweet potato a few times with a fork and then wrap each sweet potato in foil and bake for about 45 minutes to 1 hour, until potato is soft and a knife can easily move in and out. When cool, remove the peel and cut into chunks. Blend the sweet potatoes, tofu, dates, and cinnamon until smooth. Add water to reach desired consistency. Chill for 1 hour in the refrigerator, then serve.

Refrigerate for up to 2 days or freeze for up to 1 month.

Note

To add calories, add 1 teaspoon of coconut oil to each serving to provide an additional 40 calories and 4.6 grams of fat.

NUTRIENTS PER SERVING: 1 serving: 2 tablespoons • Calories: 49.3 • Total Fat: 0.4 g • Saturated Fat: 0.1 g • Protein: 1.4 g • Carbohydrates: 10.8 g • Fiber: 1.6 g • Sugar: 6.1 g • Vitamin A: 67.2 mcg • Vitamin C: 4 mg • Calcium: 22.5 mg • Iron: 0.4 mg • Potassium: 131.3 mg • Sodium: 17.7 mg • **Provides approximately 1 vegetable serving and 1 protein serving for infants 7 to 8 months.**

Mama's Chicken Soup

We do love quick and easy recipes, but for classic chicken soup we made an exception. The key is cooking the soup slowly at a low temperature to obtain the most flavor out of the vegetables and the bone in chicken, especially since we want to avoid salt for young children. We've added carrots, parsnips, a sweet red bell pepper and corn to give this soup a sweet flavor to appeal to young babies. This soup is perfect alone or poured over cooked whole-wheat pastina or quinoa. | MAKES ABOUT 20 CUPS

Place chicken into a large 8-quart pot. Cover the chicken with approximately 3 quarts (or 12 cups) of water. Bring to a rolling boil and then immediately lower to a simmer. Cook covered for 2½ hours. With a spoon, skim off the foam that accumulates at the surface, every half hour or so. Add all the vegetables to the pot and bring back to a simmer (make sure only at a simmer so as to avoid the broth boiling off). Cook for 3½ to 4 hours and let cool. Once cool enough to handle, remove the red pepper, corn, parsley, dill, and garlic from the pot. Discard all. For extra flavor, squeeze the garlic cloves from the bulb into the soup and mix in. Cut up the remaining vegetables into bite-sized pieces and add back into pot. Remove all the chicken and discard skin. Shred chicken, being careful to remove all the bones, and place back into pot. Add the onion powder, optional salt and pepper to season. Puree the soup with chicken and veggies until desired consistency is reached and serve over pastina.

Refrigerate for up to 2 days or freeze for up to 2 months.

Note

To add calories, add 1 tablespoon of Parmesan cheese to each serving to provide an additional 30 calories, 2 grams protein, and 2 grams fat.

3 quarts of water, 12 cups

1 whole chicken, cut in 8ths (about 3-4 pounds)

4 small turnips, peeled and cut into 2 inch cubes

4 medium parsnips, peeled and cut into 2 inch cubes

1 large onion, peeled and quartered

7 medium carrots, peeled and cut into 2 inch cubes

1 medium red bell pepper halved, and seeded

1 corn on the cob, husk removed

1 bunch of fresh dill

1 bunch fresh parsley

1 whole head of garlic, top trimmed ¼ inch to expose the cloves.

1½ teaspoons onion powder

salt and pepper to taste

Prep time: 20 minutes

Cook time: 6 hours

Excellent source for 7- to 8-month-olds of protein and vitamins B_{12} and K.

Good source for 7- to 8-month-olds of vitamin A, folate, potassium, and zinc.

NUTRIENTS PER SERVING: 1 serving: ⅓ cup soup served with 1.5 tablespoons whole-wheat pastina • Calories: 56.5 • Total Fat: 1.7 g • Saturated Fat: 0.5 g • Protein: 4 g • Carbohydrates: 6.7 g • Fiber: 1.1 g • Sugar: 1.2 g • Vitamin A: 81.1 mcg • Vitamin B_{12}: 0.1 mcg • Vitamin K: 2.2 mcg • Calcium: 12.4 mg • Folate: 12.9 mcg • Iron: 0.4 mg • Potassium: 100.2 mg • Sodium: 17.5 mg • Zinc: 0.4 mg • **Provides approximately 1 carbohydrate serving, 1 protein serving, and 1 vegetable serving for infants 7 to 8 months.**

Real Life Parenting

Even though Janet was slightly reluctant to try foods that were less bland for both of her kids, to her surprise, both Sid and Annie loved strong flavors and spices like curry and even a bit of hot pepper!

Dina also found the same with her two daughters. When Evie went on a chicken strike, Dina mixed the pureed chicken with some garlic powder and a dash of pepper, and Evie's strike was quickly over. Julia, however, never liked the "spicier" spices and as soon as they would hit her tongue, she would immediately spit out the food. Dina learned to adapt food to her taste by adding the sweeter spices, such as cinnamon, to her chicken or a touch of vanilla to her yogurt. Chances are if you don't like eating your baby's food, your baby won't like eating it either, so we recommend making it tasty by adding spices!

Chapter Four

~~~~~~

9 to 12 Months

In chapter four, we will discuss your 9- to 12-month-old baby and answer questions about what a typical diet consists of, when to start fingers foods, choking hazards, and transitioning to whole milk. We will also address common medical concerns such as diarrhea, dehydration, anemia, and food allergies, as it pertains to these ages.

Expected Developmental Milestones

We love our children at every stage, but we must admit, this is one of our favorite periods! Your once-little baby has transformed into a small person with a big personality and strong will. Motorwise, your 9-month-old will be pulling up to stand. If you haven't already, lower the crib mattress and baby-proof the house. Your child will be sitting up well without support and possibly crawling, although for many crawling is not a developmental milestone, and some babies will just pull themselves up, start to walk, and bypass crawling altogether. Many babies will be cruising or walking while holding on to objects like the couch. In addition, they will likely be throwing (food and toys will definitely be all over the floor) and will have fine motor skills, such as an immature pincer grasp, that will then evolve into a mature pincer grasp by the end of this period (picking up small objects more precisely between thumb and second finger). Socially, your baby will delight in games of peek-a-boo and pat-a-cake, will wave good-bye, clap, and may show signs of stranger anxiety.

Language skills include tons of babbling (ma-ma, da-da, but not specifically to mom or dad), while cognitively your baby will start to explore, learn his/her name and what "no" means (typically there will be a light of understanding in their eyes when you say "no," followed by a devilish smile as they continue do to what they want to do). Babies will learn that objects still exist even when they are out of sight. This is called object permanence and corresponds with the development of separation anxiety (your baby will start to understand that when you are not with him/her, you are somewhere else, and will want to be with you!).

Your child turning 1 is an exciting milestone and you should truly be proud of how much you have accomplished during this year. So happy birthday to your little one and congratulations to you! By a year, motor skills may include standing on his/her own for a few seconds, walking unassisted, putting objects in and out of a container, and voluntarily releasing objects, and having a mature pincer grasp. Socially, your child will maintain eye contact, prefers to be around familiar people, cries when their favorite people leave, may not like being around strangers, and will start to test boundaries.

Cognitively, your child is exploring, may follow a simple command when you gesture, and may imitate your actions. Language skills bring first words like mama and dada, specifically now to mom and dad, and your child may also say one or two other words and point to grab your attention.

Developmental Milestones for 9–12 Months

AGE	MOTOR AND VISUAL SKILLS	SOCIAL SKILLS	COGNITIVE/LANGUAGE
9 months	Pulls up, sits up without support, may crawl, cruises, throws, holds own bottle and will have an immature pincer grasp.	Plays peek-a-boo and pat-a-cake, waves good-bye, claps, and may show signs of stranger and separation anxiety.	Babbles (may say "mama" and "dada" but usually not specifically), explores, understands more such as knows name, what "no" means, learns object permanence.
12 months	Stands for a few seconds, may walk unassisted, puts objects in and out of a container, and voluntarily releases objects, and develops a mature pincer grasp. Vision fully formed to adult level.	Maintains eye contact, prefers to be around familiar people and cries when they leave, starts to test parental boundaries, may not like being around strangers, may show fear in particular circumstances.	May say "mama" and "dada" with specific meaning as well as one or two other words, points to grab your attention, or may make gestures, such as shaking head "no." Explores objects and may use them correctly (puts phone to ear), follows a simple command when you gesture, will come to you when called, and may imitate your actions.

FEEDING SKILLS

Able to mash food with gums and tongue (does not need teeth to eat) and moves food from side to side in mouth, wants to feed self by picking up food with pincer grasp (later likes to attempt to spoon-feed self) able to drink from a sippy cup and then a straw cup more easily.

Basic Nutritional Guidelines

Between 9 and 12 months of age, your child will likely be ready to eat chunkier foods and finger foods. We will discuss in this section how to know when to begin finger foods, what are choking hazard for babies, when and how to switch to whole milk, and if your growing baby can overfeed.

Range of Calories per Day	
AGE	**CALORIES PER DAY***
9–12 Months	Males: 793–844
	Females: 717–768

*This range of calories is an estimate based on the average child. Your child may require more or less calories.

Adapted from USDA Food and Nutrition Service's Infant Nutrition and Feeding Guide for Use in the WIC and CSF Programs.

Typical Menu for 9 to 10 Months

Morning: Breastfeeding or 7 to 8 ounces breast milk or formula

Breakfast: 1 to 2 tablespoons cereal plus 1 to 2 tablespoons fruit

Mid-morning: Breastfeeding or 7 to 8 ounces breast milk or formula

Lunch: 1 to 2 tablespoons vegetable plus 1 to 2 tablespoons soft, cooked, bread, cereal, or starch

Late afternoon: Breastfeeding or 7 to 8 ounces breast milk or formula

Dinner: 1 to 2 tablespoons meat, other protein, or dairy plus 1 to 2 tablespoons vegetables

Bedtime: Breastfeeding or 7 to 8 ounces breast milk or formula

Totals:

Milk intake: 3 to 4 feeds; 24 to 32 ounces

Grains: 2 to 3 servings (1 serving: 1 to 2 tablespoons)

Fruits and vegetables: 2 to 3 servings (1 serving: 1 to 2 tablespoons)

Proteins: 1 serving (1 serving: 1 to 2 tablespoons)

Typical Menu for 10 to 12 Months

Morning: Breastfeeding or 7 to 8 ounces breast milk or formula

Breakfast: 1 to 2 tablespoons cereal plus 2 to 3 tablespoons fruit

Mid-morning: Breastfeeding or 7 to 8 ounces breast milk or formula

Snack: 2 to 3 tablespoons fruit

Lunch: $1/2$ to 1 ounce meat, other protein, or dairy plus 2 to 3 tablespoons vegetables plus 1 to 2 tablespoons cereal or soft bread

Late afternoon: Breastfeeding or 7 to 8 ounces breast milk or formula

Snack: 1 to 2 tablespoons cereal or bread

Dinner: $^1/_2$ to 1 ounce meat, other protein, or dairy plus 2 to 3 tablespoons vegetables plus 1 to 2 tablespoons cereal or soft bread

Bedtime: Breastfeeding or 7 to 8 ounces breast milk or formula

Totals:

Milk intake: 3 to 4 servings, 24 to 32 ounces of formula/breast milk until 1 year old and then 16 to max of 24 ounces of whole milk.

Grains: 4 servings (1 serving: 1 to 2 tablespoons)

Fruits and vegetables: 4 servings (1 serving: 2 to 3 tablespoons)

Proteins: 2 servings (1 serving: $^1/_2$ to 1 ounce)

Finger Foods

At around 8 to 9 months, most children should be developmentally ready to eat finger foods. In this section, we discuss when and how to introduce finger foods and provide information on how to avoid choking hazards.

How do I know my baby is ready for finger foods?

When your baby is about 8 or 9 months old, he/she will be able to sit unassisted, will develop the immature "pincer grasp" (might grab a fistful instead of one Cheerio!), allowing him/her to pick up small pieces of food, and will be able to place food in his/her own mouth. Stage 3 foods, which are chunkier in texture, and finger foods can now be started. Babies do not need teeth to start finger foods, since they will be able to mash food with their gums. Parents often worry about their babies choking on small bites of food and feel like they should crush

Use of Pouches

Like most parents, we love the convenience of pouches! However, it is important to offer your child foods of different consistencies and textures so they can develop good oral-motor coordination. We recommend limiting the use of pouches and offering them more age-appropriate table foods. Remember, pouches are still just purees even though they are packaged differently.

As always, we recommend reading labels, too, since well-intentioned parents may use the pouches to get in extra veggies, but the labeled veggie may only be a small part of the pouch's ingredients.

up their child's first Cheerio until it's only Cheerio dust! We understand the fear of choking, but babies really want to feed themselves at this age and are ready for table food. In addition, eating table food is important in the development of oral-motor muscles and in helping with language development.

What are some good finger foods?

Foods that you can easily mash between your lips can be given to babies and should be about the size of a pea, or approximately ¼ inch. Examples include pieces of whole-grain macaroni, whole wheat pancakes, cheese, soft fruits and veggies, scrambled eggs, and small bits of meatball, tofu or meatloaf, poultry, low-mercury fish, or veggie burgers. After 1 year, you can feed your baby anything that you are eating, including honey and whole milk, while avoiding choking hazards such as foods that are cylindrical and can block a child's airway (see page 129 for a list of potential choking hazards).

What are good snack foods for my baby to eat?

Great snack options are always soft, ripe, small pieces of fruit like bananas, avocados, blueberries, melon, pears, peaches, and strawberries. Other good choices include unsweetened applesauce, plain whole-milk yogurt, small pieces of shredded cheese, no added salt whole-fat cottage cheese or ricotta cheese sweetened with fruit or cinnamon, small pieces of whole-wheat or bran muffins, whole wheat crackers with a thin smear of peanut butter, and plain Cheerios. Remember that serving sizes are small at this age and are usually around 1 to 3 tablespoons for each food, or the size of the baby's palm.

My baby loves Cheerios. I know I can't feed honey to my baby until after 1 year, but can I give food that contains honey, like Honey Nut Cheerios?

The spores of *C. botulinum* are resistant to heat and may survive even after several hours of boiling. There is a potential risk, then, for infants given processed foods containing honey like Honey Nut Cheerios and honey graham crackers to develop botulism. Therefore, it is better to play it safe and avoid honey-containing foods until after 1 year of age.

What are common choking hazards?

Children most frequently choke on hard candy, followed by other candy, large pieces of meat, bones, raw or hard pieces of fruits and vegetables, seeds, nuts, shells, snacks (such as chips, pretzels, popcorn, biscuits, cookies, and crackers), hot dogs, and bread.

Choking

Choking occurs when food or objects block the airway, causing your child not to be able to cough (or have a weak cough), cry, talk (if older), or breathe. If your child has a strong cough (or is talking, if older), then encourage them to cough to try to expel the object on their own. It is always safest to call 9-1-1 if you are concerned your child is unable to expel a piece of food and is choking. We also recommend all parents or caregivers to take a CPR class to be prepared for these situations.

Common Choking Hazards

- Hard candy
- Large pieces of meat (sausages or meat sticks)
- Bones (in poultry and fish)
- Raw, hard fruits and veggies like carrots and apples
- Seeds, nuts, shells
- Chips, pretzels, popcorn
- Hot dogs (food most commonly associated with fatal choking)
- Grapes
- Marshmallows
- Chunks of peanut butter
- Chunks of cheese, such as melted string cheese
- Cherry tomatoes or other small tomatoes
- Gum

Other foods that may be choking hazards include grapes, marshmallows, melted cheese, chunks of nut butter, and gum. We advise parents to avoid choking risks by cutting fruits, veggies, and meat lengthwise into thin strips and then into small pieces, about the size of a pea. Cut hot dogs lengthwise into thin strips and then into small quarters and likewise, cut grapes and small tomatoes into quarters as well (see image, page 130). Avoid some foods all together like nuts and hard candy until your pediatrician says it is safe to do so and your child can chew them well. Babies should only be offered a few pieces of food at a time, to avoid them placing too much in their mouths at once. Children should always be supervised while eating, should be sitting in their high chair at the table and never be running, playing, or lying down while eating.

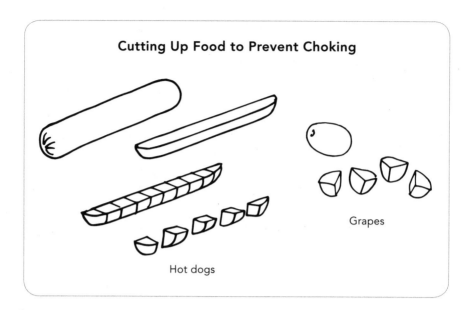

Cutting Up Food to Prevent Choking

Grapes

Hot dogs

When can I switch my baby to whole milk and how much should she have?

After a year you can switch to whole cow's milk and your baby should be taking a maximum of 24 ounces of whole milk, with a range of 16 to 24 ounces of milk a day (less than this is appropriate as long as there are other sources of calcium in the diet, please see page 155 on different milk options). Some babies love the taste, so you can offer your baby a bottle, sippy, or straw cup of whole milk and see if he/she likes it. If your baby does not initially like the taste, we recommend gradually adding the whole milk in to the bottle, sippy, or straw cup by mixing mostly breast milk or formula with an ounce of whole milk and slowly increasing to all whole milk. If your baby refuses, you can also try warming up the milk or mixing it with their favorite fruit such as strawberries or blueberries to give it a sweet added flavor. Fresh fruit is a better option than artificially flavored chocolate or strawberry powders.

My baby is always eating! Can he overfeed at this age?

Infants have a good barometer of when they are full and satiated. However, as they get older, children, like adults, may become emotional eaters and look to food when they are bored, anxious, depressed, lonely, or happy. Concerns about weight can begin as early as the preschool years, and emotional eating has a peak incidence in the early teen years, usually between 9 to 12 years of life.

Although emotional eating starts in older children, parents should help create a positive relationship with food early on. During infancy, parents should listen to cues about when a child is full, such as turning away from the nipple, decreased sucking, or falling asleep after having a full tummy. Also, bottle-fed infants may not finish the entire bottle, which is okay, and in most cases, as long as there is adequate weight gain, is completely normal. During early childhood, parents should avoid offering food as a reward or giving a toddler a sweet just to stop their crying, and parents should try to understand why and when a child is eating. Family meals should be eaten without any distractions, including television, smartphones, or tablets to prevent young children from mindlessly overeating. If you are concerned about your child's intake, speak to your pediatrician who can review your child's growth charts with you to assess whether your child is growing appropriately for his/her age.

Expected Growth

Children's weight gain will continue to increase at a similar rate as 7- to 8-month-olds. On average, they should gain weight at a rate of 1 ounce every three days and should triple their birth weight by 1 year of life. They will grow at a rate of $3/8$ of an inch per month in length and $1/4$ of an inch per month in head circumference. By 1 year of life, their head circumference increases on average by 5 inches and length by 10 inches as compared to their measurements from birth.

Medical Concerns

As your child is exploring more, going to classes, and making new baby friends, your child also might catch his/her first illness. In this section, we discuss diarrhea, its treatment, and signs of dehydration. Also during this stage, your baby will have blood drawn, probably for the first time, to look for anemia. We will discuss what anemia is and what are good foods to eat to prevent anemia. We will end with a discussion on whether to have your child tested for food allergies and the guidelines on receiving the flu vaccine if your child has an egg allergy.

Diarrhea

Diarrhea is one of the most common illnesses faced in childhood and is defined when a child passes looser and more frequent stools than normal or about three or more in a day. Acute diarrhea is often caused by viruses, but can be due to bacteria and parasites.

My baby has diarrhea. When should I call my pediatrician?

You should speak to your pediatrician if your child's diarrhea is associated with blood in the stool, the diarrhea lasts more than five to seven days, or if your child has persistent vomiting, fevers, a swollen (distended) stomach, is in pain when his/her stomach is touched, or there are any signs of dehydration (see page 134). You should also call your pediatrician if you or your child recently returned from international travel, or if your child has other chronic medical illnesses. Your pediatrician will discuss with you how to best keep your baby hydrated.

What should my child be drinking and eating if he/she has diarrhea?

For mild diarrhea, children can continue breast milk or formula feeding as usual, along with your baby's regular diet. It is usually unnecessary to change formulas, for example, to a lactose-free formula, or to restrict a child's diet. If, however, you notice your child's normal formula, which is often cow's milk–based and contains lactose, or your breast milk (lactose is also in breast milk) is upsetting your little one's tummy or making the diarrhea worse, you should talk to your pediatrician about temporarily switching to a lactose-free formula, including soy-based ones (if over a year old, then soy- or lactose-free milk). Although pediatricians may tell parents to feed their baby the BRAT diet (bananas, rice, applesauce, toast), there is no clinical data supporting its effectiveness. If your child refuses to eat the foods in the BRAT diet, it is simply better to provide your child with a diet full of age-appropriate foods, as long as he/she is able to tolerate the food.

If your child has moderate diarrhea, your pediatrician may suggest giving your baby an oral rehydration solution, such as Pedialyte, which replaces electrolytes and fluid lost with diarrhea and helps in the prevention of dehydration (please see chart, opposite, for estimated daily requirements of electrolyte solution). If your child is also vomiting, the electrolyte solution should only be given a little bit at a time. For example, start by giving one teaspoon every five to ten minutes, with a gradual increase in the amount as tolerated and not a lot at once; if your baby gulps the fluid down, it might be too much for his/her sensitive tummy to handle and he/she could vomit it right back up. It is always a good idea to have Pedialyte at home in case your child gets sick. Pedialyte and generic forms of it are available in a premixed solution, individual powder packets that can be mixed in water, or in the form of an ice-y (our personal favorite). Diluted juice such as watered-down white grape juice, which lacks sorbitol that may contribute to diarrhea, is also an option. Other fruit juices, including apple juice, contain sorbitol and more fructose than glucose (two other types of sugars) and can often cause diarrhea and are not good choices to offer your child. Your pediatrician may suggest coconut water, which is another source of electrolytes, if your child does not like the taste of the rehydration solution. It is not recommended that you make a rehydration solution on your own since it is very easy to mix the ingredients incorrectly which may be harmful to your child. It is also not recommended to give water alone, since children need to replenish electrolytes they have lost, or to give food and drinks high in sugar, like gelatin and full-strength juice, since these can make the diarrhea worse. Your child may not eat solids well during the first few days of the illness, which is okay, as long as they are drinking and have an adequate number of wet diapers. Children will start to eat solid foods again as they begin to feel better.

Estimated Electrolyte Solution Requirements by Body Weight for Mild Diarrhea

WEIGHT IN POUNDS	OUNCES OF ELECTROLYTE SOLUTION (IN 24-HOUR PERIOD)
6–7	16
7–11	23
11–22	40
22–26	44
26–33	51
33–40	61

Adapted from AAP Caring for Your Baby and Young Child, Birth to Age 5, 4th Edition.

Can I give my child medications for the diarrhea and does he/she need any special tests?

Giving your child antidiarrheal medications such as loperamide (Imodium) is not recommended. Using probiotics specifically containing Lactobacillus GG has been shown to shorten the course of mild to moderate diarrhea by one day.

In addition, your pediatrician may recommend testing your child's stool for infectious causes, especially if there is blood in the stool. Most of the time even if a bacterial cause is identified, antibiotic therapy is not indicated nor is it helpful, as the majority of the infections will resolve on their own. Antibiotics also often have their own set of side effects and can possibly make symptoms worse.

What is lethargy?

The term "lethargic" is often used incorrectly. True lethargy is an emergency and does not mean that a child is a little under the weather. It means that your child may be unresponsive, not making eye contact, limp, excessively sleepy and difficult to arouse, or very sick looking. If this describes your child, your physician should be made aware immediately. Children will often appear less active with a fever, but if your child perks up and is more active after acetaminophen or ibuprofen (after six months) is given, then likely this is not true lethargy.

Signs of Dehydration

MILD TO MODERATE	SEVERE
Thirst	Increased thirst
Decreased urine output	No urination or dark yellow urine
Mouth has no moisture and mucus Membranes and tongue are dry	Lips parched and cracked
Skin is dry	Skin is clammy
Deep set eyes	Sunken eyes
Decreased tears	No tears
Fontanelle (soft spot) flat	Fontanelle sunken
Fussiness and irritability	Lethargic (limp, not responding)
Pulse normal to slightly increased	Rapid pulse
Mild weight loss	More significant weight loss

Common Causes of Diarrhea in Infants

Infectious	Bacteria: *Salmonella*, *Shigella*, *Campylobacter*, and *Escherichia coli* Parasitic: Giardia Viral: Rotavirus, Norwalk virus
Diet	Fruit juice (prune, pear, and apple juice)
Medications	Antibiotics, certain antacids

Anemia

Anemia is when the hemoglobin, the part of the red blood cell that carries oxygen, is lower than is normal based on your child's age. It is common for your pediatrician to check a hemoglobin level between 9 months and 1 year old. The most common cause of low hemoglobin at this age is due to iron deficiency. In this section, we will discuss signs of anemia and list foods that contain good sources of iron.

My pediatrician took blood work at the 9-month or 1-year visit to check if my child is anemic. What are the symptoms of anemia?

Your pediatrician did blood work called a CBC (complete blood count), which looks at hemoglobin and red blood cells. Children with mild anemia will have no symptoms, but some signs and symptoms of more severe anemia would be pale skin, easily tired, short of breath, and a heart murmur that may be heard by your pediatrician.

What is a common cause of anemia in toddlers? What foods can I add to my child's diet that improve iron absorption?

Anemia can be caused by a variety of reasons. One common cause is nutritional, found in toddlers who do not eat iron-rich foods or who drink large amounts of milk, which fills them up so they are not eating as much iron-rich foods. There are two types of iron, heme and non-heme iron. Heme iron is from animals and is easily absorbed into the body, while non-heme iron is from plant sources and is not as easily absorbed. However, when vitamin C–rich foods are eaten together with non-heme iron-rich foods, iron absorption is improved. For example, eating lentils with broccoli (vitamin C–rich) at the same meal, will aid in non-heme iron absorption (see Broccoli-Lentil Soup, page 142). Meat, fish, and poultry also enhance non-heme iron absorption.

How much iron does my child need?

If your child is healthy, the Recommended Dietary Allowance (RDA) for iron is listed in the table on page 136. If, however, your child is found to be anemic, your pediatrician will suggest increasing iron in the diet, may recommend decreasing dairy consumption, and may place your child on a multivitamin with iron or liquid iron supplement until the anemia resolves and your baby's body replenishes his/her iron stores.

Recommended Dietary Allowance (RDA)+ for Iron for Children

AGE	IRON (MILLIGRAMS PER DAY)
0–6 months	0.27 mg per day*
7–12 months	11 mg per day
1–3 years	7 mg per day

+RDAs (Recommended Dietary Allowance) are the average daily dietary intake levels that sufficiently meet the nutrient requirements of nearly all (97 to 98%) healthy individuals in a group.
*Adequate Intake (AI) is used when there is not enough information available to list RDA.

Adapted from the USDA Dietary Reference Intakes.

Sources of Heme Iron-Rich Foods

SOURCES OF HEME IRON	AMOUNT*	MILLIGRAMS OF IRON
Clams	1 ounce	7.9
Oysters	1 ounce	1.9
Beef liver	1 ounce	1.9
Beef	1 ounce	0.8
Duck	1 ounce	0.8
Shrimp	1 ounce	0.6
Lamb	1 ounce	0.5
Light tuna	1 ounce	0.5
Poultry (dark meat)	1 ounce	0.4

Source: ESHA The Food Processor Software

Sources of Non-Heme Iron-Rich Foods

SOURCES OF NON-HEME IRON	AMOUNT*	MILLIGRAMS OF IRON
Fortified cereals	½ cup	4.6
Blackstrap molasses	1 tablespoon	2.7
Soybeans	¼ cup	2.2
Spinach	½ cup (cooked)	1.9
Lentils	¼ cup	1.7
Navy beans	¼ cup	1.1
Cashews	2 tablespoons	1.0
Refried beans	¼ cup	1.0
Kidney beans	¼ cup	0.9
White beans	¼ cup	0.9
Lima beans	¼ cup	0.9
Tomato puree	2 tablespoons	0.6
Potato with skin	½ medium	0.6
Chickpeas	¼ cup	0.5
Eggs (especially yolks)	1 large yolk	0.5
Raisins	2 tablespoons	0.4
Tofu	1 ounce	0.4
Prunes/prune juice	2 prunes	0.2

*The amounts of iron listed in these charts are only examples of high-iron foods and are not suggested serving sizes for this age group. Some foods, including whole cashews, are not recommended for this age group.

Source: ESHA The Food Processor Software

Food Allergies

In this section, we discuss if and when to have your child tested for food allergies and also review the guidelines for receiving the flu vaccine if your child has a reaction to eggs.

My 9-month-old had a rash after eating eggs. When can I have him tested for an egg allergy? What is the youngest age allergy testing can be performed, and what does testing entail?

Yes, a 9-month-old baby can definitely be tested for egg allergy. There is no age limit for allergy testing, and allergy testing is possible with most foods. Allergists have a few ways of doing allergy tests. There are skin prick (or scratch) tests, which can be done for foods, environmental allergens, and some medications. Blood samples can also be sent for allergic antibody (IgE) levels for most any food or environmental allergen (like pollen or pets).

If egg, or any new food, seems to trigger an allergic reaction in your baby (see chapter two or six for more details on food allergies), it might be reasonable to have that food (and related foods) allergy tested. You should be aware, though, that the vast majority of food allergies are to a few foods: milk, eggs, soy, wheat, peanuts, tree nuts, finned fish, shellfish, and sesame. Although egg and milk allergies are more common food allergies in infants and young children, they are often outgrown.

Extensive allergy testing is very rarely needed for young infants, even for those who may have allergic issues. It is important to restrict the tests to things that are more often culprits (like the major food allergens) or likely to be in the baby's diet at the time, or introduced very soon. It is also unhelpful to do skin tests for very obscure food allergens, like spices or to foods that are uncommon problems (most fruits, vegetables, and meats), unless the medical history suggests a specific problem with these foods. Finally, it is important to know that allergy testing does not necessarily tell the future. A baby's negative allergy test is no guarantee that a food allergy will not develop later in childhood or during adulthood. "Testing for everything," is usually not the best or most reliable way to approach diagnosing or predicting food allergies in a child.

My son has a severe allergy to peanuts. My 9-month-old daughter has never had peanut butter. Should she be tested for peanut and other food allergies?

While there is an increased risk of food allergies for siblings of children with food allergies, the expert panel that developed and updated the Guidelines for the Diagnosis and Management of Food Allergy does not recommend routine *general* food allergy testing for non-allergic younger siblings of a food-allergic child.

If, however, there is some other indication for testing your baby for food allergies (like persistent severe eczema) or if some food allergies, like milk or eggs, have already developed during the first months or year of your child's life, then it is a good idea to see an allergist. The allergist can determine whether there is sensitization present for other allergenic foods that may not have been introduced yet or that you may be nervous to feed your baby. For instance, children with cow's milk or egg allergies are more likely to be allergic to peanuts, and children with a peanut allergy are more likely to be allergic to tree nuts. Through appropriate allergy testing, an allergist can help you navigate what allergenic foods may safely be introduced next.

As previously mentioned in chapter two, there is now some evidence that we may be able to prevent peanut allergy from developing in babies who are "at risk" (but not already allergic) by introducing it into the diet before 1 year of age. We are now recommending that an evaluation specifically for peanut allergy be done for babies between 4 and 8 months of age who have persistent or moderate-to-severe eczema, other food allergies, or who are at risk. "At risk" babies may include those who have a family member (parent or sibling) with an allergy to peanuts. Avoidance of peanuts in these children may actually be counterproductive, and is associated with a higher risk of later developing a peanut allergy.

My daughter developed a rash after eating eggs. Can I still give her the flu shot?

The short answer is likely "yes." Here, though, is the longer answer and some precautions to consider. Both the injectable and nasal mist forms of the influenza vaccine contain a very tiny amount of egg protein; however, it has been shown that this is not enough to trigger an allergic reaction for the vast majority of people with egg allergy, even for those who have a very severe egg allergy. Currently, though, only the *injectable* flu vaccine is recommended for those with egg allergy. The nasal influenza vaccine (which can be given to children over 2 years) is not recommended for anybody with egg allergy or asthma; this recommendation may change in the future if more studies show that it is safe. So, unless your child has had an allergic reaction to the injectable flu vaccine itself, there is really no reason to avoid it. The yearly flu vaccine is an important childhood vaccine, as the influenza virus can cause severe sickness in babies and young children. We recommend that your child receive the influenza vaccination, even if certain precautions due to an egg allergy may be necessary.

As of the 2015–2016 flu season, the recommendations with regard to egg allergy and the flu vaccine are as follows:

- If a child has a history of an egg allergy, but is now able to eat eggs, she can receive the injectable flu vaccine.
- If a child has a history of a mild reaction (no more than several local hives) after eating eggs, she can still receive the flu vaccine as a single injection dose in the pediatrician's office, but should be observed closely for thirty minutes following immunization.
- If your child has received the influenza vaccination in prior years without any issue or reaction, she can receive it in subsequent years in the pediatrician's office.
- If a child has a more severe egg allergy, referral to an allergist may be recommended before giving the flu vaccine. The allergist will, in most cases, give the vaccine in a single dose, but will also observe the child closely for at least 30 minutes. In some cases, the allergist may choose to give the flu vaccine in a few smaller doses. Yes, that means giving several injections in order to get to the full dose.

Healthy Recipes for 9 to 12 Months

Developmentally, your baby can now pick up small pieces of food and wants to feed him/herself, making this stage a perfect time to start finger foods and foods with soft chunks. During this time, if your baby is having trouble gaining weight, when feasible, we also included suggestions on how to increase the calories in the recipe.

For these recipes, we make the claim that a recipe is a "good source" of a certain nutrient when the serving size we list meets 10 to 19 percent of the Dietary Reference Intake (DRI) for the 9 to 12 month age group. We claim a recipe is an "excellent source" of a nutrient when the serving size listed meets 20 percent or more of the DRI for the 9 to 12 month age group. Also, as there are no fiber requirements for this age, we will note which recipes contain high amounts of fiber.

Real Life Parenting

When Sebastian began to eat finger foods, Anthony noticed that he developed a rash on his cheeks. The rash was worse when he ate homemade tomato sauce. Anthony was initially concerned that Sebastian may be allergic to tomato sauce. It also happened when he first tried the Beef Veggie Bolegnese (see page 143). Sebastian really enjoyed eating these foods and he was otherwise doing well and never developed any other allergy symptoms. Anthony applied cream to Sebastian's face and offered him tomato sauce again a few days later. With the moisturizer in place, the rash did not reoccur, and Sebastian continues to enjoy pasta with tomato sauce as one of his favorite meals.

Broccoli-Lentil Soup

This hearty lentil soup is full of vegetables, protein, and fiber. It provides a soft, chunky texture for your baby to chew. In addition, broccoli not only contains fiber and iron, but it is also an excellent source of vitamin C. When vitamin C–rich foods are eaten in combination with non-heme iron-rich foods, such as lentils, iron absorption is improved. | MAKES 9½ CUPS

1 tablespoon olive oil

1 medium onion, finely chopped

2 carrots, peeled and finely chopped

2 stalks celery, finely chopped

1½ cups dry lentils

1 (15 ounce) can diced tomatoes

1 head broccoli, cut into florets (approximately 3½ cups)

2 quarts chicken broth, low sodium

½ teaspoon dried cumin

Heat the oil in a 6-quart saucepan over medium heat. Add the onions, carrots, and celery and sauté for 5 minutes, or until they begin to sweat. Add the lentils, tomatoes, broccoli, broth, and cumin and stir to combine. Cover and bring to a boil, then reduce to a simmer. Simmer for 45 minutes or until the broccoli and lentils are tender. Cool, then puree until the soup reaches the desired consistency.

Refrigerate for up to 2 days or freeze for up to 1 month.

Note

To add calories, add 1 tablespoon of Parmesan cheese to each serving to provide an additional 30 calories, 2 grams protein, and 2 grams fat.

Prep time: 20 minutes

Cook time: 50 minutes

Excellent source for 9- to 12-month-olds of protein, vitamins B_{12}, C, and K, potassium, zinc, and folate.

Good source for 9- to 12-month-olds of vitamin A, calcium, omega 3-fatty acids, and iron.

NUTRIENTS PER SERVING: 1 serving: ½ cup • Calories: 94.4 • Total Fat: 1.8 g • Saturated Fat: 0.4 g • Protein: 6.8 g • Carbohydrates: 14.5 g • Fiber: 3 g • Sugar: 1.9 g • Vitamin A: 76.4 mcg • Vitamin B_{12}: 0.1 mcg • Vitamin C: 16.2 mg • Vitamin K: 2.1 mcg • Calcium: 31.4 mg • Folate: 46.5 mcg • Iron: 1.8 mg • Omega-3 fatty acids: 0.1g • Potassium: 320.1 mg • Sodium: 74.7 mg • Zinc: 0.84 mg • **Provides approximately 2 vegetable servings and 2 protein servings for infants 9 to 12 months.**

Beef-Veggie Bolognese

This sauce will provide your baby with veggies, new spices, fiber and the perfect texture to be eating at this stage. Served over quinoa for added protein, it's an easy and complete dinner that the whole family will enjoy. | MAKES APPROXIMATELY 4½ CUPS SAUCE

Preheat oven to 400°.

Put tomatoes on a baking sheet lined with parchment paper. Roast for 25 minutes until slightly browned and shriveled.

Place onion, carrots, and celery in a food processor fitted with the blade attachment. Pulse together until finely ground but still has some texture. Add the roasted tomatoes and blend until a chunky sauce is achieved.

In a large frying pan, heat the olive oil on medium heat and sauté garlic for 2–3 minutes until slightly browned, being careful not to burn. Add the vegetable mixture and cook for 5 minutes. Add ground beef, canned tomatoes, and the oregano. Break up the meat into the sauce and simmer for 15–20 minutes until the meat is cooked through and the sauce has reduced slightly. Stir in basil and Parmesan cheese. Serve over quinoa.

Refrigerate up to 3 days or freeze up to 2 months

Note

To add calories, add in 1 tablespoon of no-salt-added ricotta cheese to provide an additional 27 calories, 1.8 grams protein, and 2 grams of fat.

1½ cups whole cherry tomatoes, (about 25 tomatoes)

1 cup coarsely chopped onion (approximately ½ medium yellow onion)

½ cup coarsely chopped celery (approximately 2 stalks celery)

½ cup coarsely chopped carrots (approximately 1 large carrot)

2 tablespoons olive oil

2 cloves garlic, minced

1 pound ground beef (80 percent lean)

2 cups canned chopped tomatoes

1 teaspoon oregano

1 tablespoons fresh basil, roughly chopped

¼ cup freshly grated Parmesan

4½ cups cooked quinoa

Prep time: 10 minutes

Cooking time: 1 hour

Excellent source for 9- to 12-month-olds of protein, vitamins B_{12} and K, and zinc.

Good source for 9- to 12-month-olds of folate and potassium.

NUTRIENTS PER SERVING: 1 serving: 2 tablespoons sauce and 2 tablespoons cooked quinoa • Calories: 75.4 • Total Fat: 3.9 g • Saturated Fat: 1.2 g • Protein: 3.6 g • Carbohydrates: 6.4 g • Fiber: 1.1 g • Sugar: 1 g • Vitamin B_{12}: 0.3 mcg • Vitamin K: 1.5 mcg • Calcium: 16 mg • Folate: 12.4 mcg • Iron: 0.7 mg • Potassium: 99.1 mg • Sodium: 52 mg • Zinc: 0.8 mg • Provides 1 protein serving, 1 carbohydrate serving, and 1 vegetable serving for infants 9–12 months.

Salmon and Sweet Potato Frittata

These frittatas are soft, easy to chew, and a great introduction to table food and fish in particular. Fish is an important source of healthy omega-3 fatty acids and protein. It is a quick meal and very tasty as breakfast, lunch, or dinner for the entire family to enjoy. | MAKES 8 SERVINGS

1 medium sweet potato, peeled and cubed

3 whole eggs

2 tablespoons whole milk

½ pound fresh salmon fillet, baked and shredded

1 tablespoon unsalted butter

Prep time: 10 minutes

Cook time: 20 minutes

Excellent source for 9- to 12-month-olds of protein, vitamins B$_{12}$ and D, omega-3 fatty acids, and potassium.

Good source for 9- to 12-month-olds of vitamins A and E, folate, and zinc.

Preheat the oven to 350°F.

Place the cubed sweet potato in a pot of boiling water. Boil for 5 minutes, or until soft. Drain and let cool.

In a bowl, whisk the eggs and milk. Stir in the cooled sweet potato and the cooked salmon.

Heat the butter in a medium nonstick, 8-inch oven-safe pan over medium heat until melted. Pour in egg-salmon mixture and cook for 2 minutes. Place the pan in the oven and continue cooking an additional 10 to 12 minutes or until the egg has set and does not jiggle.

Refrigerate for up to 2 days or freeze for up to 1 month.

Note

To add calories, add 1 teaspoon of melted butter to each serving to provide an additional 33 calories and 3.8 grams fat.

NUTRIENTS PER SERVING: 1 serving: 1/8 of recipe (1 ounce of cooked fish) • Calories: 94.6 • Total Fat: 4.9 g • Saturated Fat: 1.9 g • Protein: 8.8 g • Carbohydrates: 3.2 g • Fiber: 0.5 g • Sugar: 1.1 g • Vitamin A: 97.9 mcg • Vitamin B$_{12}$: 1.9 mcg • Vitamin D: 143.4 IU • Vitamin E: 0.5 mg • Vitamin K: 0.2 mg • Calcium: 20.6 mg • Folate 11.3 mcg • Iron: 0.5 mg • Sodium: 69 mg • Zinc: 0.4 mg • Omega-3 fatty acid: 0.4 g • Potassium: 183.6 mg • Provides approximately 1 vegetable serving and 1.5 protein servings for infants 9 to 12 months.

Pulled Apricot-Raisin Chicken

This chicken dish is pull-apart tender—a perfect table food for your 9- to 12-month-old. The apricots and raisins add sweetness to the chicken, making this dish a favorite for both toddlers and babies alike.

| MAKES 6 BONELESS CHICKEN BREASTS

Preheat the oven to 325°F.

Place the chicken in a 9 by 9-inch baking dish. Whisk the oil and orange juice together and pour over the chicken. Scatter the apricots and raisins on and around the chicken and pour in the stock so that the stock covers the entire chicken. Cover with foil and bake for 90 minutes or until fork tender. Discard the poaching liquid and pull the chicken apart with forks. Season with salt (for toddlers and adults) and pepper to taste.

Serve warm or refrigerate for up to 3 days or freeze for up to 2 months.

Note

Because chopping is often a tedious and time-consuming task for parents, particularly as little ones cause chaos in the kitchen, we find it helpful to pulse the raisins and apricots in a food processor until they are the right bite-sized portions for babies, or less than a quarter of an inch.

To add calories, add 1 teaspoon of olive oil to each serving to provide an additional 40 calories and 4.6 grams fat.

2½ pounds boneless, skinless chicken breasts (about 6 chicken breasts)

2 tablespoons olive oil

½ cup orange juice

10 dried apricots chopped (see Note)

¼ cup raisins, chopped (see Note)

1½ cups low-sodium chicken stock

Salt and pepper (optional for kids over 1 year of age)

Prep time: 5 minutes

Cook time: 90 minutes

Excellent source for 9- to 12-month-olds of protein, vitamin B_{12} and potassium.

Good source for 9- to 12-month-olds of zinc.

NUTRIENTS PER SERVING: 1 serving: ¼ chicken breast • Calories: 82.2 • Total Fat: 2.5 g • Saturated Fat: 0.5 g • Protein: 10.5 g • Carbohydrates: 4 g • Fiber: 0.4 g • Sugar: 2.4 g • Vitamin B_{12}: 0.1 mcg • Calcium: 7.1 mg • Iron: 0.3 mg • Potassium: 208.2 mg • Sodium: 60.3 mg • Zinc: 0.3 mg • **Provides approximately 2 protein servings for infants 9 to 12 months.**

Spinach-Quinoa Bites

After eating these easy-to-make homemade veggie burgers, you will definitely taste the freshness over the frozen ones. They are high in fiber and lower in sodium than most store-bought burgers. The red bell pepper, an excellent source of vitamin C, helps improve absorption of the iron found in spinach. | MAKES 9 TO 10 BURGERS

⅓ cup of quinoa, rinsed and drained

⅔ cup water

1 teaspoon of olive oil

2 cups fresh spinach leaves

½ red bell pepper, seeded and finely diced

1 large russet potato, peeled, cooked, and mashed

1 egg, beaten

1 cup shredded mozzarella cheese

⅔ cup shredded Parmesan cheese (optional)

Prep time: 10 minutes

Cook time: 45 minutes

Excellent source for 9- to 12-month-olds of protein, vitamins C and K, calcium, folate, and potassium.

Good source for 9- to 12-month-olds of vitamins B₁₂ and E, and zinc.

Bring the quinoa and water to a boil over medium heat. Cover and reduce to a simmer. Simmer for 10 minutes, then remove from the heat and let sit for another 5 minutes with the lid on. Remove the lid and fluff with a fork.

In another medium saucepan, heat the olive oil. Add the spinach and cook just until it has wilted, about 3 to 5 minutes. In a mixing bowl, mix the cooked spinach, red pepper, quinoa, potato, egg, mozzarella, and optional Parmesan cheese.

Line a baking sheet with parchment paper and preheat the oven to 350°F.

Scoop ¼ cup of the mixture at a time onto the baking sheet and flatten with a spoon, forming approximately 9 to 10 burgers. Bake for 20 to 30 minutes, or until the tops brown. Serve warm.

Refrigerate for up to 3 days or freeze for up to 1 month.

Note

To add calories, add optional Parmesan cheese to provide an additional 30 calories, 2 grams protein, and 2 grams fat.

NUTRIENTS PER SERVING: 1 serving: 1 burger • Calories: 97.9 • Total Fat: 4 g • Saturated Fat: 1.8 g • Protein: 5.7 g • Carbohydrates: 11.2 g • Fiber: 1.3 g • Sugar: 0.6 g • Vitamin A: 48 mcg • Vitamin B₁₂: 0.1 mcg • Vitamin C: 12.1 mg • Vitamin E: 0.5 mg • Vitamin K: 31.5 mcg • Calcium: 99.2 mg • Folate: 31.3 mcg • Iron: 0.7 mg • Potassium: 192.6 mg • Sodium: 86.2 mg • Zinc 0.4 mg • Provides approximately 2 servings carbohydrates, 1 serving vegetable and 1 serving protein for infants 9 to 12 months.

Chapter Five

The Toddler Years

In chapter five, we focus on the early toddler years. We discuss milk options after weaning your baby from breast milk or formula, what children should be eating at this stage, and guide parents on how to deal with picky eaters. We end this section with a discussion on common concerns such as toddler's diarrhea, potty training, and constipation.

Expected Developmental Milestones

Oh, the toddler years! Parents are often fearful of entering the "terrible twos," but we truly believe this period offers some of the most rewarding and memorable moments. Seeing the world through your toddler's wonder-filled eyes, hearing your baby say "I love you" for the very first time, and being bestowed with sloppy, random kisses when you least expect them, make us wish we could freeze this stage in time forever.

Motorwise, by around 15 months your baby should be walking by him/herself, usually with an unsteady wide-based gait. Don't worry if your baby isn't walking before 15 months—early walking is not associated with being advanced in other areas of development! Your child will likely begin to crawl up stairs, stoop to pick up objects, and walk backward. Your baby will also gain more balance and will typically learn to run, albeit stiffly, at 18 months, and with greater ease by 24 months. By 18 months, your child will begin to walk up stairs with one hand held and will be an expert at throwing objects. At 2 years of life, your toddler will walk up and down stairs independently and will begin to jump.

Socially, this stage is noted for your child developing a sense of self and independence. Your 12-month-old should maintain eye contact and will start to imitate you, and can follow commands paired with a gesture. By 15 months, your child will be able to follow simple one-step commands not accompanied by a gesture, will begin to say "no," test limits, and may start having temper tantrums. At 18 months, toddlers will be imitating common chores like sweeping and cooking, may throw more temper tantrums, and exhibit behaviors like hitting, biting, and pulling hair to seek attention (time to set consistent limits and reward good behaviors to allow the desired behavior to win out over the bad).

Language Development

Parents often worry if their 12-month-old is not saying any words yet, or has an expressive language delay (problems talking and gesturing), but there is a *wide* range for normal speech development. Children should understand more than they can say at this age. If at any time you have questions or concerns about your child's language development, or any other developmental concerns, it is important to bring them up with your pediatrician, who may recommend a hearing test or further evaluation.

Surprisingly, at 18 months, your child might also become more clingy, making them your little shadow wherever you go, and bedtime may become a battle as your child has to leave your side. By 24 months, your little one will be following more complex two-step commands, and will meet the milestone of parallel play where your child will play alongside, but not usually with, another child. Young toddlers do not often interact with each other, unless one child dares to steal the other's beloved toy, which might lead to their first fight with friends.

Developmental Milestones for Toddlers

AGE	MOTOR AND VISUAL SKILLS	SOCIAL SKILLS	COGNITIVE/ LANGUAGE
15 Months	Walks by self with an unsteady wide-based gait, crawls up stairs, stoops to pick up objects, walks backwards, builds a tower of two blocks.	Follows simple one step commands, tests limits, and may start having temper tantrums.	Says around two to six words, may say "no," jargon, able to understand more than can express, and communicates with not only words but also with pointing and gesturing.
18 Months	Gains more balance and learns to run, walks up stairs with one hand held, can scribble, use a spoon, and build tower of three blocks.	Imitates common chores, may throw more temper tantrums, and exhibits behaviors like hitting, biting, and pulling hair to seek attention, may become more clingy.	Says around seven to ten words, can say "no," jargons with words that are understandable, identifies one or more body parts. Loves to explore and has no fear.
24 months	Runs with greater ease, walks up and down stairs, throws or kicks a ball, begins to jump with two feet off the floor, can build a tower of four to six blocks.	Follows more complex two-step commands, engages in parallel play, likes being around other children but does not share easily, is possessive over toys.	Says around fifty words, and is speaking in simple two-word sentences. Uses pronouns.

FEEDING SKILLS

Makes more precise up-and-down tongue movements, is able to wean off bottle to cup, attempts feeding self with utensils, able to eat food that requires chewing, and can be offered anything you eat except choking hazards.

Your child's language will make a dramatic transition by the end of this stage. Toddlers will often say their first words around 12 to 15 months, but are able to understand much more than they can express, and will communicate with you in other ways, too, such as pointing to interesting objects and jargoning (stringing babbled words together with expression, as if they are talking in sentences). By 15 months, your baby will say around two to six words and by 18 months will say seven to ten words and jargon will include words that you understand (mature jargoning). At around 2 years of age, there is typically an explosion in language development. Your child will have a vocabulary of at least fifty words, will use pronouns, and will likely be speaking in simple two-word sentences.

Basic Nutritional Guidelines

In this section, since your toddler will transition to whole milk and everything you are eating, we will discuss a toddler's typical menu, the nutritional content of whole milk and other milk alternatives, as well as the difference between various carbohydrates and organic and nonorganic snacks. We will also review how much your toddler should consume of salt, sugar, fat, and other foods such as eggs and fish.

How much should a toddler be eating, calorie-wise and also in frequency?
Parents often are concerned if their children are eating enough and serve portions that resemble the amounts that adults should be eating. In reality, small children really don't need very much food. In general, by age 2, toddlers are eating three healthy meals and two snacks a day, with the average 2-year-old boy and girl both requiring approximately 1,000 calories a day—roughly 40 calories per inch of height per day.

Range of Calories per Day	
AGE	CALORIES PER DAY*
1–2 Years	900–1,000
2–3 Years	Sedentary 1,000–1,200 Moderately active or active 1,000 to 1,400

*This range of calories is an estimate based on the average child. Your child may require more or less calories, depending on a variety of factors including their activity level.

Adapted from USDA Food and Nutrition Service's Infant Nutrition and Feeding Guide for Use in the WIC and CSF Programs and the USDA Dietary Guidelines for Americans 2010 and US Department of Health and Human Services.

Typical Menu for Toddlers

The menu below is a guideline for assessing appropriate intake. Intake may vary for each individual child within an age range, and also may vary each day. The best indicator that your child is eating enough food is consistent weight and height gain. See charts starting on page 220 for more details.

This menu is for 1- to 3-year-olds and includes servings. See the table on page 152 for more details.

Breakfast: 1/2 cup whole milk (1/2 dairy) plus 1/2 cup cooked oatmeal (1 grain) plus 1/2 cup pear slices (1/2 fruit)

Snack: 1/2 cup fresh apple slices (1/2 fruit) plus 1 1/2 ounces cheese (1 dairy)

Lunch: Half of a turkey sandwich on whole-grain bread (1 grain) with 1/2 ounce turkey (1/2 protein) plus 1 cup mixed green salad (1/2 vegetable) with 1 teaspoon Italian dressing (1 fat)

Snack: 2 to 3 small whole-grain crackers (1/2 grain) with 1 to 2 tablespoons hummus (1/2 protein)

Dinner: 1/2 cup quinoa (1/2 grain) plus 1 ounce baked white fish (1 protein) plus 1/2 cup cooked spinach (1/2 vegetable) sautéed in 1 teaspoon of olive oil (1 fat) plus 1/2 cup whole milk (1/2 dairy)

Water in a cup with all meals and snacks.

Totals:

Dairy: 2 to 2 1/2 cups

Grains: 2-3 servings

Fruits: 1 cup

Vegetables: 3/4 to 1 cup

Proteins: 1.5 to 2 ounces

Fats and Oils: Do not limit during 12–23 months; limit to 3 teaspoons per day for 2 to 3 years old

Miscellaneous: Desserts and sweets use sparingly.

Dried Versus Fresh Fruit

Toddlers should have 1 cup of fruit per day. A half cup of dried fruit is equivalent to 1 cup of fresh fruit, so remember to adjust the portion size when eating dried fruit. Also, choose dried fruit that is just fruit and does not contain added sugar or preservatives.

Feeding Guide for Toddlers

FOOD GROUP	12–23 MONTHS	2–3 YEARS	SERVING SUGGESTIONS	HELPFUL TIPS
Dairy	2 cups whole milk or equivalent per day	2–2½ cups low-fat (1%) or non-fat milk per day	1 cup milk = 1 cup yogurt, 1½ ounces cheese, ⅓ cup shredded cheese	May use low-fat or fat free dairy or cheese for children over 2 years Limit use of dairy products with added sweeteners (such as chocolate milk)
Grains and Starches	2 ounces per day	3 ounces per day	1 ounce = 1 slice bread, ½ cup cooked rice or pasta, 1 cup dry cereal	Choose at least half whole grain daily including whole-wheat flour, oatmeal, and brown rice Limit refined grains including white flour and white bread
Fruits	1 cup per day	1 cup per day	1 cup = 1 cup of raw or cooked fruit, ½ cup dry fruit, 1 cup fruit juice	Use fresh or frozen fruit instead of juice or canned fruit which may contain added sugar
Vegetables	¾ cup per day	1 cup per day	1 cup = 1 cup raw or cooked vegetables or 1 cup vegetable juice, 2 cups raw leafy greens	Incorporate different groups of vegetables in the diet every week including dark-green, red and orange, starchy, and beans and peas Home-prepared beans are preferred for lower sodium content. If using canned beans, drain beans from liquid and rinse in water to decrease salt content.
Proteins	1½ ounces per day	2 ounces per day	1 ounce = 1 ounce beef, poultry, or fish; ¼ cup cooked beans; 1 egg; 1 tablespoon nut butter	Aim for fish twice a week as good sources of protein and omega-3-fatty acids Choose lean meats and poultry for children over 2 years. Lean beef is at least 92% lean. Limit salami, bacon, hot dogs and cured meats
Fats/Oils	Do not limit. Low-fat products not recommended	Up to 3 teaspoons per day	1 teaspoon = 1 teaspoon oil, 1 teaspoon of butter, 1 tablespoon of sour cream	For children over 2 years, choose healthy fats like olive, canola, and sunflower oils
Miscellaneous	Limit to small amount, use sparingly	120–140 discretionary calories		These are foods that provide empty calories and no added nutrition.

Adapted from the USDA's Preschooler Daily Food Plan and Texas Children's Hospital Pediatric Reference Guide 2013, *10th edition.*

When should I introduce utensils?

Each child develops at his/her own rate, but most children will be excited to use a spoon and attempt feeding themselves at around 1 year. Babies will start off by simply dipping the spoon in their food and initially will not get much food in their mouth, but by 15 months will be able to fill the spoon more fully and actually get food into his/her mouth on a more regular basis. By 18 months, your baby should be able to use a spoon and even a fork with more ease. We recommend starting off with foods that a toddler can more easily pick up themselves with a spoon, which will create less frustration, such as oatmeal or mashed potatoes. Examples of foods that are easier to pick up with a fork are pieces of macaroni and pancake.

Are most toddlers eating enough fruits?

Toddlers should be eating 1 cup of fruit per day. According to a recent study, only 40 percent of children over 2 years old met this requirement. The most popular fruit consumed is apple followed by citrus juices, bananas, melons, berries, and citrus fruit. A little over half of all fruit consumed by toddlers is in the form of whole fruit, while 100 percent fruit juices make up about 1/3 of fruit consumption. Remember it is always better to offer your toddler a variety of fresh fruit (and limit the use of fruit juices) so that they meet the recommended daily intake!

Milk and Dairy Products

Now that your child is over 1 year, you can switch from formula or breast milk to whole cow's milk, or a milk alternative. For breastfed babies, this switch can happen any time after a year, as breastfeeding may continue as desired by the mom and child.

After 1 year of age, milk is no longer providing the majority of nutrients in your child's diet, and it is now a beverage to go with their meals instead of a meal itself. It is, however, still an important source of protein, fat, calcium, vitamins, and minerals.

> ## Cow's Milk and Stool Pattern
> Your child's stool may change when whole cow's milk is introduced. Sometimes they become looser, and at other times they may be harder and more difficult to pass. As your child adapts to the introduction of cow's milk, it may be helpful to add foods to the diet that will normalize your child's stool pattern.

Whole cow's milk is the most popular choice to transition to after breast milk or formula. It tends to be a good nutritional complement to a typical toddler's diet, and if your child has no reason to avoid cow's milk, it's our preferred choice. There are, however, many alternatives to whole cow's milk, particularly if your child has an allergy to cow's milk, simply does not like to drink it, or if you prefer not to give this type of milk. Some of these include soy, almond, coconut, and rice milks. If you use one of these alternatives, look for "enriched" products fortified with calcium, vitamin D, and often other vitamins and minerals. Also be aware that nondairy milks typically contain less protein, fat, and calories than whole milk (see page 155). Every brand varies, and there are even ingredient variations within the same brand, so check labels carefully to find the product that packs the most nutrition. If your child is a good eater and receives nutrients found in cow's milk from other dietary sources, it's likely fine to use an alternative.

Should I give my child a toddler formula instead of cow's milk?
Many toddler formulas have been introduced in the last several years to try and bridge the nutritional gap between infant formulas and toddler diets. Toddler formulas are nutritionally similar to infant formulas with added calcium, and some brands contain omega-3 supplementation and prebiotics. The cost of these specialty toddler formulas tends to be higher than infant formulas and whole milk. For the most part, we think these formulas are unnecessary for the toddler with a normal (even selective) diet, who drinks cow's milk. In the majority of children with prolonged picky eating, a pediatric multivitamin may suffice to give the additional vitamins and minerals.

When can I change to low-fat milk?
Dietary fat at this age is particularly important for brain development. Most children will continue on whole cow's milk until age 2, but in some cases, your

pediatrician or dietitian may recommend starting reduced-fat (2 percent) milk after one year of age. The American Academy of Pediatrics (AAP) recommends starting reduced-fat (2 percent) milk between 12 months and 2 years of age in

Comparison of Whole Cow's Milk and Popular Alternatives (per cup)

	CALORIES	PROTEIN (GRAMS)	FAT (GRAMS)	CALCIUM (MG)	VITAMIN D (IU)
Whole cow's milk (vitamin D fortified)	149	8	8	276	124
Whole goat's milk (fortified with folic acid)	140	8	7	300	100
Vanilla soy milk	100	6	3.5	450	120
Vanilla almond milk	80	1	2.5	450	100
Vanilla rice milk	130	1	2.5	300	100
Vanilla coconut milk	80	0	4.5	100	120
Toddler formula	160	6	6	270	100

Comparison of Whole and Reduced-Fat Cow's Milk (per cup)

	CALORIES	PROTEIN (GRAMS)	FAT (GRAMS)	CALCIUM (MG)	VITAMIN D (IU)
Whole cow's milk (vitamin D fortified)	149	8	8	276	124
2% milk	122	8	5	293	120
1% milk	102	8	2	305	117
Fat-free milk	83	8	0	299	115

children *at risk* of being overweight, or whose families have a history of obesity, heart disease, or high cholesterol.

In all other children, it is recommended to continue whole milk until your child is 2 years old. After age 2, your child could switch to low-fat (1 percent) or nonfat milk. However, these recommendations, like other recommendations in medicine, may change in the future as more research is done on this topic, and it is always best to speak with your pediatrician before you change your child's diet.

I want to give my child soy milk, but is too much soy milk unhealthy for my toddler?

There is a lot of conflicting evidence on the pros and cons of soy products, such as tofu, edamame, and soy milk, and no solid research on the effects of soy consumption in children. Most studies have been done in animals who may not process soy in the same way children do. The debate stems from soy containing isoflavones or phytoestrogens, which are chemically similar to estrogens. Soy has been linked to lowering the risk of osteoporosis, heart disease, and breast cancer, but because it resembles estrogen, it has also been thought to cause infertility. The AAP states that there is no conclusive evidence in animal or human studies that soy will have a negative effect on development, immune, thyroid, or reproductive functions. The Harvard School of Public Health also believes there is still much to be learned on the effects of soy and makes a more conservative recommendation to limit soy consumption to less than two servings per day. We agree that more studies in children are needed before a definite recommendation can be made, but as many cultures have been safely eating soy products for years, soy is likely safe to consume in appropriate serving sizes.

Now that my child has been weaned off of the bottle, he/she refuses to drink milk. What should I do?

Toddlers are creatures of habit and like their set routines, so it is no surprise that they are resistant to the thought of drinking milk from a cup after transitioning off of their beloved bottle. Their bottle is familiar and sucking provides comfort. If at first your child refuses to drink milk from a cup, keep offering it to him/her and don't give up. It might help to offer it in a favorite sippy, straw, or "big girl or boy" regular cup. It may also help to slowly introduce the new milk by offering a cup mixed with one-quarter milk and three-quarters formula or breast milk, and gradually working your way up to all milk over a few days. Try warming up the milk, especially if your child is not used to refrigerated milk, or mixing it with a favorite fruit (crushed up strawberries or blueberries with milk tastes delicious!). Often, with a little patience, the milk strike will soon pass. If the protests continue, don't worry, and simply offer other sources of vitamin D and calcium (see below). Remember, from 12 to 23 months, toddlers only need two cups of whole milk or milk products per day.

If my child doesn't drink a lot of milk, should I be worried about vitamin D deficiency? What are other good sources of vitamin D to give my baby besides milk?

If your toddler isn't eating a well-balanced diet rich in vitamin D foods, you should talk to your pediatrician about starting a supplement. Some

Sources of Vitamin D

FOOD	SERVING	VITAMIN D (IU)
Swiss cheese	1 ounce	6
Ready-to-eat cereal (fortified)	¾ to 1 cup	40
Egg yolk	1 large	41
Margarine (fortified)	1 tablespoon	60
Orange juice (fortified, may vary)	½ cup	68.5
Tuna fish (canned in water, drained)	1 ounce	51.3
Yogurt (fortified)	6 ounces	80
Salmon (sockeye) cooked	1 ounce	149

Adapted from the NIH's Vitamin D Fact Sheet

Rickets

Rickets is a form of extreme vitamin D deficiency that we rarely encounter now due to increased use of vitamin supplements in babies and vitamin D fortification of milk and other foods. Rickets causes the bones to become weak and more prone to be deformed and fractured.

examples of foods rich in vitamin D include milk, cheese, egg yolks, salmon, sardines, tuna, and foods that are fortified with vitamin D like cereals, orange juice, margarine, and yogurt. Choose a plain baby yogurt, which is usually fortified with vitamin D, instead of adult whole fat yogurts, which are usually not fortified.

Children who are more at risk for vitamin D deficiency include babies who are born prematurely and require more calcium and phosphorus, children who eat an extremely limited diet (not your average picky eater), or children with chronic medical conditions such as chronic kidney disease, liver disease, cystic fibrosis, or seizure disorders (antiseizure medications may lead to the breakdown of vitamin D). Darker-skinned children, and children living in areas of high levels of air pollution or decreased exposure to sunlight, are also at higher risk for vitamin D deficiency.

My toddler loves carbs. Is there really a difference between white, whole-wheat, and multigrain breads?

Carbohydrates are an important part of a toddler's diet, although all carbs are not created equally. Try to provide at least half of carbohydrates from whole-grain sources. Here is the breakdown:

- Whole-grain foods contain the naturally occurring parts of the whole-grain seed (bran, germ, and endosperm). The bran and germ contain vitamins, minerals, and fiber. These foods are more nutrient dense than their refined counterparts, are more filling, and may reduce the risk of diabetes and heart disease. Look for foods that list whole grains on the ingredient list, including whole-grain wheat flour, bulgur, and oatmeal.
- Foods made from white flour and other refined carbohydrates have the bran and germ removed during the refinement process. Thus, the majority of nutrients and fiber are removed. Eat less of these foods, including refined white breads, white rice, and white pastas.
- Multigrain products are made from a variety of grains (for example oat, wheat, rye); however, unless the product specifies that it is whole grain, it may be made of refined flour and missing nutrients that are found in the bran and germ of whole grains seeds.

Is it better to give my toddler organic snacks?

There is a common misconception that because a snack food item is organic, that it is always a healthy choice. It's a good idea to look deeper, even when you see "organic" labeling on a package, since organic junk food is still junk food.

Many organic snacks and their nonorganic counterparts are in fact very similar in terms of nutrient profile, and would be on our list of "sometimes foods." For example, take an organic and nonorganic cheddar snack cracker. Both contain approximately 150 calories, 5 to7 grams of fat, 250 milligrams of sodium (approximately 17 percent of daily recommended intake for toddlers), and less than 1 gram of fiber per serving. Not our top choice for an everyday snack food! Some snacks that are always a good idea would include fruits; vegetables; low-sugar, reduced fat yogurts (reduced fat if over 2 years); and high-fiber, low-sugar cereals.

When your child occasionally indulges on a less healthy snack, there are some benefits of choosing organic, if your budget allows for it. Organic snacks contain no artificial colors, flavors, or synthetic preservatives. They are produced without antibiotics or synthetic hormones, may contain fewer pesticides, and are not produced with genetically modified ingredients.

My child is over 2. How much salt, sugar, and fat can be in his/her diet?

Salt: Although your child's kidneys can now handle a larger amount of salt, it's best to limit the amount in your child's diet as it may reduce the risk for high blood pressure and other diseases as your child ages. The recommended daily intake for sodium is less than 1,500 milligrams, with an adequate intake of approximately 1,000 milligrams, or about half a teaspoon, for 1- to 3-year-olds. This isn't much, and your child can easily meet his/her needs without adding extra salt in the diet. Be sure to check labels and steer clear of big salt offenders often found in processed foods like certain canned soups and beans, sauces, frozen dinners, lunch meat, and condiments.

Sugar: It's a good idea to limit added sugars, from foods like cakes, cookies, sodas, and fruit drinks, which provide empty (nonnutritive calories), and can lead to health problems and chronic diseases when consumed in excess. Sugar can also be found hidden in "healthier" snacks too like flavored yogurts, flavored milks, cereals, granola bars, cereal bars, muffins, and dried fruit based snacks. Parents often ask us if it's better to choose cane sugar or more natural sweeteners like honey, maple syrup, or agave nectar, instead of high fructose corn syrup, but studies so far have found little evidence that high fructose corn syrup differs from other sweeteners. Honey and maple syrup tote a slight advantage to cane sugar or high fructose corn syrup, in that they contain more antioxidants. However, the risk of added dietary sugar still outweighs the benefits provided by these antioxidants.

The USDA groups all the above sweeteners together and it gives a general guideline recommending a limit of empty calories that should be consumed daily. For 2- to 3-year-olds, it is between 120 and 140 calories or less, and for 4- to 8-year-olds, it is 120 calories or less. Other sources are slightly more liberal, recommending up to 165 to 170 calories for 2- to 3-year-olds and 170 to 195 calories for 4- to 8-year-olds. Be sure to read labels and provide tasty healthy snacks like fruit whenever possible. It is not recommended that children consume artificial sweeteners since the long-term effects for children are unknown.

Fat: Up until the age of 2, fat should not be limited in a child's diet to promote healthy growth and brain development. The AAP recommends parents to offer foods with less saturated fat and to avoid trans fat for children ages 2 to 5 years old. Saturated fats mostly come from animal sources and include fatty meats, poultry skin, lard, butter, cream, and full-fat cheeses. Although we may recommend adding some of these foods to your child's diet if he/she is not gaining weight appropriately, these changes should only be made after discussing with your pediatrician and dietitian. Trans fats will be labeled as partially hydrogenated or hydrogenated vegetable oils and are found in many baked goods including cakes, frozen pies and ready-to-use frostings. In 2015, the FDA announced that trans fat in the form of artificial partially hydrogenated oils will need to be removed from food products within three years as they are no longer "generally recognized as safe." Trans fats that are naturally produced in meat and dairy products, however, can still be present.

The American Heart Association recommends keeping total fat intake between 30 and 35 percent of calories for children ages 2 to 3 years. To achieve these goals, switch to lower fat dairy products, use leaner cuts of meat, avoid high-fat cooking methods like frying, trim excess meat fat, and remove poultry skin. It is recommended that fats come from healthy sources of polyunsaturated and monounsaturated fatty acids. Examples would be fish, nuts, and vegetable oils like olive and canola.

My child only wants to eat eggs every day. How often can I give eggs?

We often get this question, but this is a hard one to answer since there are no guidelines for children! Eggs contain many nutrients such as vitamin A,

B vitamins, and phosphorous, and can be part of a healthy diet. Recent studies in healthy adults demonstrate that eating up to one egg per day does not likely contribute to the risk of coronary artery disease or stroke. Since children need healthy fats and eggs are such a great source of protein, we believe that one egg a day should also be safe for healthy children. Egg whites or products like Egg Beaters are a good alternative if your child asks for more eggs, or you bake with eggs frequently. Since the egg yolk contains high levels of cholesterol and saturated fat, if you have a strong family history of high cholesterol and cardiac disease, you should discuss this further with your pediatrician because in this case you may need to limit eggs in your child's diet.

How often should I be giving fish, and what is the best type of fish to eat?

Fish is touted as a good protein source, with healthy omega-3 fatty acids and low saturated fat. However, there are some risks of eating fish that may be contaminated with mercury, a compound that can have adverse health effects on a young child's developing nervous system.

It is recommended that young children completely avoid fish that contain the highest levels of mercury, including king mackerel, swordfish, shark, and tilefish, and to also limit the amount of albacore tuna to, at most, one serving size every week. Most experts agree that the benefits of eating safer fish outweigh the risks. Some safer choices include salmon, shrimp, cod, catfish, clams, light tuna, flatfish, scallops, fish sticks, and pollock. These safer fish can be eaten in two to three age-appropriate servings per week (serving size is approximately $1^1/_2$ ounces per day for a 1- to 2-year-old, and 2 ounces per day for a 2- to 3-year-old) and should always be cooked thoroughly to avoid the risk of food poisoning.

Picky Eaters

During the toddler years, as children are gaining autonomy, they often test their new independence by eating or not eating the meal you have prepared for them. It is completely normal for your toddler to eat a bowl of a favorite food on Monday, push it away on Wednesday, and ask for a second helping of it again on Friday. As long as your child is growing and developing well, there is no reason to be alarmed at these feeding behaviors. In fact, they are completely normal and the more parents stress and push their children to eat, the more amplified these behaviors may become.

In this section, we will describe tips on feeding your picky toddler as well as review available nutritional supplements and when they are truly needed. We will also help differentiate the picky eater who is developing and growing well from a child who may not be eating sufficient calories and may need further evaluation.

Any tips to help my picky eater?

Some tips that may be helpful for picky eaters include:

- Minimize distractions at mealtimes such as television and tablets.
- Avoid using food as a reward, for example, promising toddlers if they eat their veggies, they will get a dessert, because it makes the dessert appear more desirable than the healthy food.
- Involve your child in food preparation to spark interest in the meal or have them go food shopping with you. Pick a color day, for example, on a red day eat beets, strawberries, and watermelon.
- Invite your toddler's friend over for a meal. Often children will eat what their friend is eating (a little positive peer pressure). Parents often say their child eats everything at day care and is only picky at home!
- Serve meals and snacks in a routine way, preferably at a table with others, and avoid snacks or sweetened caloric beverages, such as juices and sodas (which are never needed in a child's diet), between those times.
- Make food interesting: use cookie cutters, dipping sauces, muffin trays or bite-sized portions (see Chicken-Vegetable Meatballs in Sweet and Sour Sauce on page 173 and mini Vegetable Frittata on page 52), kebabs, colorful plates, or natural food coloring. Try offering the same food in different ways and textures: steamed, roasted, with a favorite dipping sauce, smeared with a food your child likes, or have your toddler make his/her own fun food creations. As an alternative to cookies and sugary

desserts, Dina's daughter created "Julia's cinnamon, vanilla, and banana yogurt smoothie" and loves asking for it as a special treat after dinner.

- Encourage your child to try new foods many times. Don't give up or become frustrated if it doesn't happen the first, second, or even tenth time! Offer small portions of the new food with old favorites. Over time kids may grow to like foods that they initially avoided.
- Never lie to your toddler or mask the food that they do not like. Toddlers are very smart and will catch on.
- Make meals enjoyable, not stressful!
- Model the behavior you would like to see in your children. If you expect your kids to eat a plate of veggies, you should also serve yourself veggies as well.
- There is no reason to become a short-order cook at mealtimes for your picky eater since this may further encourage bad behavior. Offer two healthy choices, and if rejected, just try again tomorrow. Toddlers will be *okay* and will not starve if they skip a meal once in a while. Remember, what they don't like today, they might like tomorrow, and it is often more realistic to judge how well they are eating over a week rather than a single day. Remember picky eating is usually just a passing phase—get creative and have fun with it!

There are many books written on the difficulties of feeding behaviors. A great and thorough resource for this topic is Ellyn Satter, a registered dietitian and family therapist (www.ellynsatterinstitute.org). Ellyn pioneered the evidence-based "Division of Responsibility" model, which is built on the idea that children innately know how to regulate food intake. This model emphasizes that parents should decide the what, when, and where of feeding. This includes maintaining meal and snack structure, limiting inappropriate snacking, choosing healthy food, modeling healthy eating, making mealtimes pleasant, and teaching the child appropriate mealtime behavior. Parents then give their child the autonomy by trusting their child to choose from what is available at those eating times, and eat as much or little as he/she desires.

Since my toddler is such a picky eater, should I start him on a multivitamin or another supplement?

For toddlers who eat a full range of foods, a daily vitamin is usually not necessary. Even a typically picky toddler is probably getting sufficient amounts of the nutrients they need. You may want to talk to your pediatrician, however, about vitamin and mineral supplements if your toddler:

- Has a *very* restricted diet and avoids one or more food groups due to refusal, allergy, or a strict vegetarian diet;
- Does not drink fluoridated water;
- Has a chronic medical condition that may impair absorption of nutrients; or
- Is not gaining weight as expected for his/her age.

If needed, a multivitamin is usually sufficient. However, your child may need an iron supplement if he/she has iron-deficiency anemia, a fluoride supplement if you do not live in an area with fluoridated water, or a vitamin D supplement if your child is not taking in the required amount of vitamin D.

Here are other popular supplements parents may wonder about:

Vitamin- and mineral-fortified drinks: There are many fortified drinks especially marketed to healthy kids to do things like help your kids grow or balance out a diet. Unless they are specifically recommended by your health care professional, we don't recommend use of these drinks, as they can be high in calories, and may replace nutritious foods in the diet. Examples include Pediasure, Pediasure Sidekicks, Boost Kid Essentials, and Pediasmart.

Fish oils: It is recommended that kids eat fish rich in omega-3 fatty acids such as salmon, trout, and herring, to help prevent heart disease, and possibly improve health by promoting brain development and lowering the risk of asthma. There are no established recommendations or guidelines for dosing fish oil supplements in children. Research on supplements are inconclusive as to the effectiveness, and brands may be poorly regulated and may contain inconsistent amounts of omega-3s.

Use of Probiotics for Medical Conditions

CONDITION	EFFECTIVE PROBIOTIC
Antibiotic-associated diarrhea	S. boulardii, Lactobacillus GG
Mild to moderate acute diarrhea	Lactobacillus GG
Atopic dermatitis (eczema)	Lactobacillus GG, L. paracasei, combo of L. reuteri and L. rhamnosus
Infantile colic	Lactobacillus reuteri

Probiotics: This is another popular supplement thought to increase beneficial bacteria in the gastrointestinal tract. Current evidence shows some benefit to using probiotics to lessen the severity of diarrhea during a stomach bug, prevent diarrhea associated with antibiotic use, and help with eczema. There is also some evidence that it can help decrease the symptoms of infantile colic. See chart on page 164 for specific details. Probiotics are felt to be generally safe, but there is no evidence for widespread supplement use in all children.

Expected Growth

Toddlers will start to gain weight at a slightly slower rate after their first birthday. Their weight will increase by approximately 1 ounce every five days, or 1 pound every three to four months. They will continue to grow at this rate until approximately 10 years of life. Between the first and second year of life, they will grow at a rate of $^3/_8$ inch per month in height or 5 inches per year. After 2 years of life, their height will increase by approximately 2 to $2^1/_2$ inches per year.

Medical Concerns

In this section, we discuss common medical concerns in toddlerhood, such as toddler's diarrhea and constipation that may occur as you begin to potty train your toddler. Since autism spectrum disorders may be diagnosed during the toddler years, we also address the special topics of whether a gluten-free diet and allergy testing is helpful for children with autism spectrum disorders

Diarrhea

Diarrhea can happen for a variety of reasons. The most likely cause of chronic diarrhea in this age group is chronic, nonspecific diarrhea, also known as toddler's diarrhea.

What is toddler's diarrhea?

Toddler's diarrhea presents typically in children between 6 months and 3 years of age. The diagnosis is made in children who have at least a three-week history of four to ten large, watery, nonbloody, and nonmucousy bowel movements daily. It is also common to see undigested food in the stool. Stools occur only during waking hours. The first stool of the day is usually the most formed and they become softer and looser throughout the day. Toddler's diarrhea is not typically associated with abdominal pain or other gastrointestinal symptoms, such as vomiting, weight loss, or poor weight gain.

The cause of toddler's diarrhea is primarily due to a high carbohydrate, low fat diet. High intake of carbohydrates, found in fruit juices, may increase the water content of stool, while low fat causes the food to move more quickly through the intestines.

Treatment of toddler's diarrhea requires dietary changes and reassurance, since the diarrhea will typically resolve on its own by 5 years old. Though diarrhea may be inconvenient and require frequent cleanups, it has no negative long-term consequences for your child. Diet changes include increasing dietary fiber and fat intake and decreasing juice intake, sport drinks, and other sources of fructose (the sugar found in fruit and fruit juices) and sorbitol (the sugar found in many dried fruits, fruit juices such as apple juice, regular fruits such as plums, prunes, and cherries, as well as sugar-free candies, gum, and other diet food). Sometimes the only diet change that may be needed is switching from low-fat milk to whole-fat milk, since increasing fat in the diet slows down stool transit time. With diet changes, symptoms of diarrhea usually improve within one to two days. Please ensure that your child is still getting adequate calories and fluid and maintaining a well-balanced diet. Antidiarrheal medications are not typically useful or recommended.

If your child has significant gastrointestinal symptoms such as vomiting, poor weight gain, or abdominal pain, your physician may recommend further testing, including stool studies and blood tests to evaluate for potential medical conditions such as an allergy, celiac disease, malabsorption, lactose intolerance, or inflammatory bowel disease. Stool tests may also help identify a chronic infection such as parasites.

Constipation and Potty Training

Constipation is a change in bowel movement frequency and consistency. At this age, both diet and behavioral control during potty training can lead to the presence, recurrence, or persistence of constipation. In this section,we will discuss how to know when your child is ready to potty train, tips for potty training, and what to do if your child becomes constipated.

How do I know if my child is ready to potty train?

Most children show an interest in potty training between 18 months to 2 years old, but the timing could be later and should never be rushed. It's always important to follow your child's cues. Potty training may take a lot of time and requires even more patience! If your child does the following, it is likely that he/she is ready to start potty training:

- Imitates your behavior
- Puts things where they belong
- Demonstrates independence by saying "no"
- Walks to the potty and sits on the potty
- States his/her need to urinate or defecate before going in the diaper

Tips for Potty Training

- Follow your child's lead and make sure he/she is interested in potty training. Never force it!
- Get a potty chair and have your child become familiar with it. For instance, encourage your child to sit on it, for as long as he/she feels comfortable, fully clothed once a day for a few days and then try it with the clothes off. You can use distractions like reading a book or singing a song. This will help him/her to relax. Some children like to have the potty in the bathroom while others prefer it be located elsewhere in the house.
- Show your child what the potty is used for by taking a stool from a soiled diaper and placing it in the potty.
- Some children prefer to potty on a "grown-up" toilet instead of their own potty chair. In this case, use a fun potty seat over the toilet bowl and also a foot stool: this will help your child more effectively push with his/her feet firmly planted and not dangling in the air.
- Make potty training fun—use sticker charts or small rewards, use lots of praise or encouragement.
- Resist pressures from others and rely on your family's, and, most importantly, your child's readiness.
- Do not start toilet training when your child is experiencing a change in his/her life, like a new day care, new sibling, recently moving, or illness as this may lead to a normal regression of stooling patterns.
- Potty training is an individual process! Most kids are successful between 3 and 3½ years old. For some children, the process may be longer, but it will eventually be successful.

I'm potty training my toddler, and now my child refuses to poop and is becoming constipated. What do I do?

If your child is having fewer bowel movements or ones that are hard and painful to pass, reassess to make sure that he/she is ready to potty train. If your toddler is demonstrating refusal to toilet train and is becoming constipated, a break in toilet training for at least a few weeks is recommended. Reinitiation of toilet training should not resume until regular bowel movements have been reestablished. Your child may be withholding stool for a variety of reasons, such as hard stools, rectal fissures, or emotional stress, and you may need to hold off on potty training until he/she is ready. If your toddler had hard stools before or is experiencing pain with stooling, it may be important to address the underlying constipation by starting with diet changes, including an increase in fiber. At this age, it is recommended that your child consume approximately 19 grams of fiber per day. You may use prune or pear juice or pureed pears or prunes, which can help make the stools softer and potty training easier (see prune pop recipe on page 97). Sometimes stool softeners recommended by your doctor may also be needed.

Autism Spectrum Disorder and Diet

Autism spectrum disorders (ASD) are being diagnosed with increased frequency. According to the CDC, the diagnosis is made in approximately 1 out of every 68 children in the United States, with boys nearly five times more frequently affected than girls. Gastrointestinal symptoms such as abdominal pain, gastroesophageal reflux, constipation, and diarrhea are more common in children with ASD as well. Diet changes are sometimes made due to the belief that food sensitivities may play a role in the behavioral, social, and cognitive concerns in children with ASD. We, therefore, will discuss here gluten-related disorders and allergy testing in these children.

My child has autism spectrum disorder. Should I avoid gluten or casein?

Parents may perceive benefits from a gluten-free diet and a casein-free diet, but evidence of these diets' impact on behavior is inconclusive. Therefore, we do not recommend avoiding gluten, unless your child has also been diagnosed with celiac disease or a gluten sensitivity. Likewise, there is no need to avoid casein unless your child has a milk allergy or sensitivity.

Due to selective eating behaviors associated with autism spectrum disorders, many of these children have a limited diet. Restricting a child's diet further, when the diet is already limited, may lead to nutritional deficiencies. The type and severity of the deficiency depend on how limited the child's diet is. Diagnoses of vitamin deficiencies may be delayed since they are not typically observed in the United States. We have seen children with autism with extremely restricted diets who present with a variety of vitamin deficiencies such as scurvy (vitamin C deficiency), rickets (vitamin D deficiency), and beri-beri (vitamin B_1 deficiency). If your child has an ASD and a limited diet, we recommend close monitoring of your child's weight and height by their pediatrician and would consider a referral to a registered dietitian and pediatric gastroenterologist to ensure your child's optimal growth.

My child has ASD or another behavior problem. Should I have my toddler tested for food allergies?

Feeding children who have developmental and behavioral disorders can be very difficult, as these children often have very picky eating behaviors and strong aversions to certain food textures, consistencies, and flavors. It is not uncommon for parents of children with autism spectrum disorders, developmental delays, or behavioral issues to see an allergist and want their child to be evaluated for food allergies. In recent years, there has been much discussion and debate about whether some behaviors may involve inflammation caused by food allergies or intolerances. The words "allergy" and "intolerance" are often interchanged (incorrectly) in these discussions, making the conversation somewhat confusing.

As discussed in chapter two, IgE-mediated food allergies can cause many symptoms. These symptoms are rarely subtle, and often cause immediate, and sometimes severe, allergic reactions. A child's behavior can also change during an allergic reaction, but this is not something that is sustained once the allergic reaction is over, and ongoing behavioral or developmental problems are not symptoms of IgE-mediated food allergies. Thus, without clinical suspicion of IgE-mediated food allergy, allergy testing (skin prick tests and specific food IgE levels) is not recommended in the evaluation or management of behavioral and developmental issues.

This is not to say that children with behavioral and developmental disorders cannot also have classical food allergies. In fact, this does occur, and presents special challenges for parents and caregivers. Children with autism spectrum disorders may not be able to verbalize or communicate when they are having acute allergic symptoms. Food allergies, however, are not a known underlying cause for autism spectrum disorder or other developmental or behavioral disorders.

Any child also can have an intolerance or sensitivity to certain foods. Food intolerances are not mediated by the immune system. Intolerances generally manifest with some digestive symptoms (for example, gassiness, bloating, and diarrhea, which occur in lactose intolerance), and do not present solely with behavioral issues or developmental delays.

Besides lactose and fructose intolerances (for which objective clinical tests are available), there really are few proven diagnostic tests for food intolerance. Nonetheless, some practitioners may prescribe special diets and dietary supplements (and sometimes intravenous vitamin infusions) or order costly tests for children who have ASD or other developmental and behavioral issues. These tests and diets, however, may not be FDA-approved and to date, these alternative modalities have not been shown to aid in the diagnosis of food allergies or food intolerance.

As there are currently no medical treatments for autism spectrum disorders and other developmental and behavioral disorders, parents frequently turn to alternative therapies in an attempt to help their children with often very challenging symptoms. We recognize that it is from a place of love and concern that parents will pursue any means possible (as long as there is no perceived harm or risk) to give their children the best care and opportunities in every realm. Still, we do recommend that you be extremely cautious if you do decide to pursue alternative test modalities and treatments. Please make sure you keep your child's doctor informed of any suspicion of food intolerance or allergy, as well as of any testing that is done, dietary changes you make, or supplements that you give your child.

Healthy Recipes for Toddlers

Your little baby has turned into an independent toddler and can now eat everything you are eating, making meals an enjoyable family experience. We are big fans of letting toddlers help you cook, making food fun for toddlers to eat, and letting them know what they are eating, so that healthy eating habits are forged early on. With this said, we are also realistic and recognize that "sometimes" snacks and meals are also a part of childhood.

For these recipes, we make the claim that a recipe is a "good source" of a certain nutrient when the serving size we list meets 10 to 19 percent of the Dietary Reference Intake (DRI) for ages 1 to 3 years. We claim a recipe is an "excellent source" of a nutrient when the serving size listed meets 20 percent or more of the DRI for ages 1 to 3 years. Prior to this age, there are no established guidelines for fiber. However, in this section, we will include fiber as an excellent or good source, as the fiber requirement at this age is 19 grams per day.

Eggplant-Zucchini Lasagna

Toddlers are known for loving a diet full of carbs and cheese, so our first toddler recipe is a healthy twist on a classic lasagna. Here we give them some of what they like to eat, but also what we love by packing this favorite full of veggies!

| MAKES ONE 9 BY 13-INCH CASSEROLE (20 SERVINGS)

1 large or 2 small eggplants, peeled and cut in ¼-inch rounds

2 large zucchinis, cut in ¼-inch rounds

1 tablespoon olive oil, plus more for brushing

Salt and pepper

8 ounces full-fat ricotta cheese

1 large egg, beaten

1 teaspoon dried basil

10 ounces frozen chopped spinach, thawed, drained, and water squeezed out (about 1 cup)

1 pound ground mixed white and dark chicken (see Note)

4 cups marinara sauce

1 cup shredded mozzarella

1 cup shredded Parmesan

10 whole-wheat lasagna noodles, cooked

Prep time: 20 minutes

Cook time: 40 minutes

Excellent source for toddlers of protein, fiber, vitamins A, B$_{12}$, C, E, and K, calcium, folate, iron, omega-3 fatty acids, and zinc.

Good source for toddlers of potassium.

Preheat the oven to 400°F.

Place the eggplant and zucchini slices on parchment-lined cookie sheets and brush olive oil on both sides. Sprinkle with salt and pepper and then roast for 15 to 20 minutes.

In a bowl, combine the ricotta, egg, dried basil, and spinach.

Heat 1 tablespoon olive oil in a saucepan over medium heat and add the ground chicken. Cook until brown and no pink is left in the center, about 10 minutes. Combine the cooked chicken and marinara sauce in a medium bowl.

Spread a thin layer of marinara sauce with the chicken along the bottom of a 9 by-13-inch baking pan, followed by a layer of lasagna noodles (about 5 noodles), a layer of the ricotta mixture, the eggplant slices, a layer of sauce, and another layer of the ricotta mixture. Sprinkle half of the mozzarella and Parmesan on top. Add another thin layer of sauce and then the zucchini slices. Finish with a layer of the remaining noodles, sauce, and top with the remaining mozzarella and Parmesan. Bake uncovered for 20 minutes or until bubbly and slightly brown on top.

Refrigerate for up to 3 days or freeze for up to 2 months

Note

We use mixed dark and white meat ground chicken in this section since toddlers under 2 need a full fat diet. Feel free to substitute white ground meat if you prefer.

NUTRIENTS PER SERVING: 1 serving: 2-by-3-inch piece • Calories: 189 • Total Fat: 8.2 g • Saturated Fat: 3.3 g • Protein: 12.5 g • Carbohydrates: 17.4 g • Fiber: 4.7 g • Sugar: 5.5 g • Vitamin A: 125.4 mcg • Vitamin B$_{12}$: 0.4 mcg • Vitamin C: 8.1 mg • Vitamin E: 2.1 mg • Vitamin K: 71.5 mcg • Calcium: 148.8 mg • Folate: 41.8 mcg • Iron: 1.6 mg • Omega-3: 0.19 g • Potassium: 583.2 mg • Sodium: 367.2 mg • Zinc: 1.1 mg • Provides approximately 1 carbohydrate serving, 1 protein serving, 1 vegetable serving, and ½ dairy serving for children 1 to 3 years.

Chicken-Vegetable Meatballs in Sweet and Sour Sauce

Toddlers love their independence and will, therefore, enjoy having their own individual, bite-sized foods (no sharing required!). We've created a meal that parents can also feel good about feeding their kids since the meatballs have added vegetables. | MAKES 30 MEATBALLS

To make the meatballs, heat 2 tablespoons olive oil in a medium pot over medium-high heat. Sauté the red pepper, mushrooms, and onion until softened, 5 to 6 minutes. Place the vegetables in a large mixing bowl and let cool slightly. Add the chicken, egg, bread crumbs, paprika, onion powder, salt, cumin, parsley, and remaining olive oil to the mixing bowl. Mix just until incorporated. Set aside while you prepare the sauce.

To make the sauce, place all the sauce ingredients plus ½ cup water into the same medium pot. Mix well and bring to a simmer.

Form the meatballs by rolling balls about the size of a golf ball and placing them into the pot with the simmering sauce. Continue with remaining mixture until you've made about 30 meatballs. Cover the pot and simmer for 1 hour, stirring occasionally.

Refrigerate for up to 3 days or freeze for up to 2 months

Note

This recipe can also be made using zucchini in place of the mushrooms if your child isn't a mushroom lover. Grate ¾ cup fresh zucchini (about 1 large zucchini). Place it in 2 layers of paper towel and thoroughly squeeze out excess water. Place on a cutting board and roughly chop it to achieve a very small dice.

MEATBALLS

4 tablespoons olive oil

½ red bell pepper, diced

3 to 4 baby bella mushrooms, finely diced (see Note)

½ red onion, finely diced

1½ pounds mixed white and dark ground chicken

1 egg, whisked

½ cup whole-wheat bread crumbs

2 teaspoons paprika

1 teaspoon onion powder

1 teaspoon salt

¼ teaspoon ground cumin

2 tablespoons fresh parsley, finely chopped

SAUCE

2 cups crushed tomatoes

3 tablespoons apple cider vinegar

2 tablespoons lemon juice

2 tablespoons maple syrup

Prep time: 20 minutes

Cook Time: 1 hour

Excellent source for toddlers of protein, vitamins B₁₂, C, E, and K, and zinc.

Good source for toddlers of iron, omega-3 fatty acids, and potassium.

NUTRIENTS PER SERVING: 1 serving: 2 meatballs • Calories: 136 • Total Fat: 8.0 g • Saturated Fat: 1.7 g • Protein: 9.5 g • Carbohydrates: 7.3 g • Fiber: 1.2 g • Sugar: 3.8 g • Vitamin B₁₂: 0.3 mcg • Vitamin C: 9.8 mg • Vitamin E: 1.2 mg • Vitamin K: 10.9 mg • Calcium: 21.7 mg • Iron: 1.1 mg • Omega-3: 0.08 g • Potassium: 382.8 mg • Sodium: 236.6 mg • Zinc: 0.9 mg • **Provides approximately 1½ protein servings and ½ vegetable serving for children 1 to 3 years.**

Sunflower Seed Butter and Fruit Quesadilla

We grew up on peanut butter and jelly sandwiches, a classic kid favorite. Many toddlers, however, have a peanut or tree nut allergy or attend school or day care where they need to bring in peanut-free lunches that can last in their backpack for several hours. Enter the sunflower seed butter and fruit quesadilla, which is a healthier version of the usual PB & J sandwich, substituting fresh fruit for the jelly. | SERVES 2

1 whole-wheat tortilla or slice whole-wheat bread

2 tablespoons sunflower seed butter, may substitute almond or peanut butter

1 banana, thinly sliced

5 grapes, thinly sliced

Toast the tortilla in the oven or toaster oven. Spread the sunflower seed butter on the tortilla and add the banana and grapes to half of the tortilla. Fold the tortilla or bread in half. Cut into bite-size pieces.

Refrigerate for up to 1 day.

Prep time: 5 minutes

Excellent source for toddlers of protein, fiber, vitamins C and E, folate, and zinc.

Good source for toddlers of iron and potassium.

NUTRIENTS PER SERVING: 1 serving: ½ quesadilla made with sunflower seed butter • Calories: 219.7 • Total Fat: 10.3 g • Saturated Fat: 1.3 g • Protein: 5.5 g • Carbohydrates: 29.4 g • Fiber: 4 g • Sugar: 11.3 g • Vitamin C: 6 mg • Vitamin E: 3.7 mg • Calcium: 14.4 mg • Folate: 50 mcg • Iron: 0.9 mcg • Potassium: 326.8 mg • Sodium: 213.8 mg • Zinc: 0.9 mg • Provides approximately 1 protein serving, 1 carbohydrate serving, and ½ fruit serving for children 1 to 3 years.

Chicken Chili

Packed with vitamins, protein, and fiber, chili is the complete package and the ultimate one-pot meal when served on top of brown rice. | MAKES 8 CUPS

In a medium pot, heat olive oil on medium heat. Add the chicken, celery, and onion and cook until the chicken is no longer pink inside and is cooked through. Stir in the tomato paste, tomatoes, broth, tomato sauce, beans, garlic, chili powder, cumin, and paprika, and bring to a boil. Reduce the heat and simmer uncovered for about 30 minutes. Season with salt and pepper to taste. Stir in the spinach and cook for 10 minutes, or until the spinach is wilted and tender. Serve over ½ cup of cooked brown rice per serving.

Refrigerate for up to 3 days or freeze for up to 2 months.

Note

To cut down on cooking time, you can dice the celery and onion in a food processor. Also, if your toddler doesn't like eating tomatoes or spicy foods, you can omit the can of diced tomato or chili powder.

To add calories, add 1 tablespoon of sour cream per serving to provide additional 23.2 calories, 0.3 grams protein, and 2.4 grams fat, or add 1 tablespoon of cheddar cheese per serving to provide additional 28.5 calories, 1.8 grams protein, and 2.3 grams fat.

1 tablespoon olive oil

½ pound mixed white and dark ground chicken

1 celery stalk, diced (see Note)

½ medium yellow onion, diced (see Note)

2 tablespoons tomato paste

1 (15 ounce) can diced tomatoes

2 cups low-sodium chicken broth

1 (15 ounce) can tomato sauce (optional, see Note)

1 (15 ounce) can kidney beans

2 teaspoons garlic, minced

1 tablespoon chili powder (optional, see Note)

1 teaspoon ground cumin

1 teaspoon paprika

Salt and pepper

2 cups spinach, chopped

8 cups cooked brown rice

Prep time: 10 minutes

Cook time: 50 minutes

Excellent source for toddlers of protein, fiber, vitamins B$_{12}$, C, and K, iron, and zinc.

Good source for toddlers of vitamin E and potassium.

NUTRIENTS PER SERVING: 1 serving: ½ cup chili with ½ cup brown rice • Calories: 220.7 • Total Fat: 5.3 g • Saturated Fat: 1.2 g • Protein: 11.9 g • Carbohydrates: 30.9 g • Fiber: 4.2 g • Sugar: 2.5 g • Vitamin B$_{12}$: 0.2 mcg • Vitamin C: 6.9 mg • Vitamin E: 0.7 mg • Vitamin K: 18.6 mcg • Calcium: 46 mg • Iron: 1.7 mg • Potassium: 469.5 mg • Sodium: 290.3 mg • Zinc: 1.3 mg • **Provides approximately 2 protein servings, 1 carbohydrate serving, and ½ vegetable serving for children 1 to 3 years.**

Ricotta Cinnamon Pancakes

Pancakes are a toddler staple—great not only for breakfast but also for a portable lunch and for "breakfast for dinner" days, too. We love this hearty pancake recipe because there is no need for maple syrup, since the sweetness is already built in with the honey. | MAKES 30 PANCAKES

1 cup whole-wheat flour

1 teaspoon baking powder

¼ teaspoon baking soda

¼ teaspoon salt

1 teaspoon ground cinnamon

1 egg, beaten

1 cup whole milk

¼ cup whole ricotta cheese

½ teaspoon vanilla extract

¼ cup honey

Unsalted butter, for greasing

Toppings (blueberries, chopped strawberries, or chocolate chips, optional)

Prep time: 10 minutes

Cook time: 20 minutes

Excellent source for toddlers of protein, vitamins A and B₁₂, and zinc.

Good source for toddlers of fiber, calcium, folate, iron, and omega-3 fatty acids.

Whisk the flour, baking powder, baking soda, salt, and cinnamon in a bowl until combined. In a separate bowl, whisk the egg, milk, ricotta, vanilla, and honey. Mix the dry ingredients into the wet ingredients until just combined; it is okay if the batter is clumpy as long as no dry ingredients are visible.

Melt 1 tablespoon of butter at a time in a large frying pan or griddle over medium heat. When the butter is hot, measure 1 tablespoon of the batter for each pancake. Sprinkle 1 teaspoon of optional toppings over the top. Cook for about 2 minutes per side, flipping when the edges start to bubble and the sides of the pancake are golden.

Refrigerate for up to 3 days and freeze for up to 1 month.

Note

To add calories, add 1 teaspoon of butter per serving to provide an additional 34 calories, 0.3 grams protein, and 3.8 grams fat.

NUTRIENTS PER SERVING: 1 serving: 5 pancakes without toppings • Calories: 186.1 • Total Fat: 5.9 g • Saturated Fat: 3.2 g • Protein: 6.3 g • Carbohydrates: 28.9 g • Sugar: 12.8 g • Fiber: 2.4 g • Vitamin A: 60.8 mcg • Vitamin B: 0.3 mcg • Iron: 1 mg • Calcium: 100.8 mg • Folate: 17.5 mcg • Omega-3 fatty acid: 0.1 g • Sodium: 281.6 mg • Zinc: 0.9 mg • **Provides approximately 1½ servings carbohydrates, ¼ serving dairy, and ¼ serving protein for children 1 to 3 years.**

Panko Fish Sticks

Made from fresh, unprocessed fish, these fish sticks pack a satisfying crunch you expect when biting into these childhood favorites. White fish, like tilapia, has a mild flavor and is an excellent source of protein and good source of omega-3 fatty acids. | MAKES 8 SERVINGS

Preheat the oven to 400°F. Line a baking sheet with parchment paper and spray with cooking spray.

Set three bowls in a row, one filled with the flour, one with the eggs, and one with the bread crumbs. Sprinkle the fish with salt and pepper. Place the fish in the flour bowl and cover both sides, then dip in the egg mixture, and coat the fish in panko bread crumbs.

Place the fish on the prepared baking sheet and bake for 10 to 15 minutes, or until the fish is completely cooked through.

Refrigerate for up to 3 days or freeze for up to 1 month.

Note

If you prefer not to use cooking spray, brush fish sticks with olive oil.

½ cup of all-purpose flour

2 eggs, beaten

1 cup panko bread crumbs

¾ pound skinless white fish (tilapia, flounder, or perch), cut into about 24 pieces

Salt and pepper

Prep time: 15 minutes

Cook time: 10 to 15 minutes

Excellent source for toddlers of protein, vitamin B_{12}, and folate.

Good source for toddlers of vitamin D, iron, omega-3 fatty acids, and zinc.

NUTRIENTS PER SERVING: 1 serving: 3 nuggets • Calories: 121.4 • Total Fat: 2.2 g • Saturated Fat: 0.7 g • Protein: 11.9 g • Carbohydrates: 13.4 g • Fiber: 1.2 g • Sugar: 0.3 g • Vitamin B_{12} 0.8 mcg • Vitamin D: 63 IU • Calcium: 37.7 mg • Folate: 40.1 mg • Iron: 1.2 mg • Omega-3 fatty acid: 0.1 g • Sodium: 201.6 mg • Zinc: 0.4 mg • **Provides approximately 1½ protein servings and ¼ carbohydrate serving for children 1 to 3 years.**

Zucchini-Apple Muffins

Sometimes a little bit of creativity goes a long way in feeding picky toddlers! We often find that toddlers love eating muffins since they can easily feed themselves and muffins resemble their much beloved dessert, the cupcake. Place these fiber- and protein-filled muffins in their favorite cupcake liner and serve them for an on-the-go breakfast or snack. | MAKES 20 REGULAR MUFFINS

3 eggs, beaten

¼ cup vegetable oil

½ cup honey

½ cup unsweetened applesauce

1 medium zucchini, grated

2 medium red apples, peeled, cored, and grated

1½ cups whole oats, finely ground in food processor

1½ cups whole-wheat flour

1½ teaspoons baking soda

¼ teaspoon baking powder

½ teaspoon salt

½ teaspoon ground cinnamon

¼ cup raisins or dried cranberries (optional)

Prep time: 15 minutes

Cook time: 25 minutes or 12 minutes for mini

Excellent source for toddlers of protein.

Good source for toddlers of fiber, iron, vitamins C and E, and zinc.

Preheat the oven to 325°F.

Mix together the eggs, oil, honey, and applesauce in a large bowl. Mix in the zucchini and apples, until incorporated. In a separate medium bowl, mix together the oat flour, whole-wheat flour, baking soda, baking powder, salt, and cinnamon. Combine the dry ingredients into the wet ingredients. Fold in the optional raisins or cranberries and mix just until blended. Line cupcake tins with 20 cupcake liners and fill with ¼ cup of batter each. Bake for 25 minutes, or until the tops are golden brown. Cool for 10 minutes.

Refrigerate for up to 2 days or freeze for up to 1 month.

Note

Use an ice cream scoop to measure out perfect muffins.

To add calories, spread on 1 tablespoon of ricotta cheese per serving to provide an additional 27 calories, 1.8 grams of protein, and 2 grams of fat.

If you prefer to make mini muffins, we recommend halving the recipe to yield 40 mini muffins. Line a mini muffin pan with liners. Fill each liner with 1 tablespoon of batter and bake for about 12 minutes, or until the tops are golden brown. Cool for 10 minutes.

NUTRIENTS PER SERVING: 1 serving: 1 regular muffin or 4 mini muffins • Calories: 125.6 • Total Fat: 4.3 g • Saturated Fat: 0.7 g • Protein: 3.1 g • Carbohydrates: 20.6 g • Fiber: 2 g • Sugar: 9.5 g • Vitamin C: 2.5 mg • Vitamin E: 0.8 mg • Calcium: 12.3 mg • Iron: 0.8 mg • Sodium: 172.4 mg • Zinc: 0.4 mg • Provides approximately 1½ carbohydrate serving, ⅛ fruit serving, and ⅛ vegetable serving for children 1 to 3 years.

Brown Rice, Broccoli, and Chicken Casserole

We fondly remember eating casseroles ourselves during family meals and wanted to include a more nutritious version of this comfort food. We again played off of toddlers' love of cheese and carbs, but added in a lean protein and a veggie to transform this into a healthier childhood favorite. | MAKES ONE 9 BY 13-INCH CASSEROLE

Preheat the oven to 375°F.

In a large bowl, mix together the rice and chopped broccoli. Mix in ¾ cup of the mozzarella, ¾ cup of the cheddar, and the Muenster. Let the cheese melt slightly. Add the chicken, sour cream, mustard, basil, and garlic powder and mix well.

Spray a 9 by 13-inch baking dish with cooking spray and pour the mixture in, flattening out slightly. Top with the remaining ¼ cup mozzarella and ¼ cup cheddar and cook uncovered for 20 to 25 minutes until golden and bubbly. Let cool slightly and serve warm.

Refrigerate for up to 3 days or freeze for up to 1 month.

2 cups of brown rice, to yield approximately 6 cups cooked rice (still hot)

3½ cups broccoli florets, finely chopped

1 cup shredded mozzarella cheese

1 cup shredded cheddar cheese

6 ounces Muenster cheese, diced

2 (4-ounce) cooked boneless, skinless chicken breasts, cut into ¼ inch cubes

1 cup sour cream

2 tablespoons Dijon mustard

½ teaspoon dried basil

1 teaspoon garlic powder

Prep time: 15 minutes

Cook time: 70 minutes

Excellent source for toddlers of protein, vitamins A, B_{12}, and C, calcium, and zinc.

Good source for toddlers of folate and omega-3 fatty acids.

NUTRIENTS PER SERVING: 1 serving: ¾ cup or 2-by-3-inch serving • Calories: 196.3 • Total Fat: 9.4 g • Saturated Fat: 5.4 g • Protein: 10.3 g • Carbohydrates: 17.6 g • Fiber: 1.7 g • Sugar: 0.8 g • Vitamin A: 96.6 mcg • Vitamin B_{12}: 0.4 mcg • Vitamin C: 13.1 mg • Calcium: 171.3 mg • Folate: 16.7 mcg • Iron: 0.6 mg • Omega-3 fatty acid: 0.1 g • Sodium: 207.8 mg • Zinc: 1.3 mg • **Provides approximately 1 carbohydrate serving, ½ dairy serving, ½ protein serving, and ¼ vegetable serving for children ages 1 to 3 years.**

Almond Butter Bites

Toddlers love to snack and should be eating one to two healthy snacks a day, giving them plenty of energy for their active days. They love bite-sized handheld snacks that make it easy to feed themselves, since everything is now about "me do it." They also love anything that resembles what their favorite grown-up is eating, so both of you can enjoy this home-made nut and fruit bar together. | MAKES 20 BARS

1 cup almonds

1 cup dates, pitted

1 cup apricots

½ cup almond butter

1 teaspoon vanilla extract

Prep time: 10 minutes

Cook time: 15 minutes

Excellent source for toddlers of protein and vitamin E.

Good source for toddlers of fiber, iron, and zinc.

Preheat the oven to 350°F.

Spread the almonds on a parchment-lined baking sheet. Toast the almonds for 10 to 15 minutes, shaking the pan occasionally to ensure they don't burn. Set them aside to cool for about 5 minutes.

In a food processor, chop the almonds until they turn into the consistency of coarse flour. Add the dates and pulse a few more times to finely chop. Add the apricots, almond butter, and vanilla and pulse until the mixture is a smooth doughlike consistency and does not contain any large pieces of dates or apricots. Flatten the mixture into an 8 by 8-inch parchment-lined baking pan. Refrigerate or freeze for 1 to 2 hours and then carefully cut into 20 bars.

Keep the bars stored in an airtight container in the refrigerator for up to 1 week or in the freezer for up to 1 month.

Real Life Parenting

When Anthony made this recipe for the first time, he quickly learned how to make almond butter. If you accidentally chop the almonds too long in the food processor, you will make the most delicious almond butter, so make sure to stop grinding the almonds once they are coarsely ground!

NUTRIENTS PER SERVING: 1 serving: 1 bar • Calories: 113.2 • Total Fat: 7.2 g • Saturated Fat: 0.7 g • Protein: 3.1 g • Carbohydrates: 10.8 g • Fiber: 2.3 g • Sugar: 6.4 g • Vitamin E: 3.2 mg • Calcium: 51 mg • Iron: 0.8 mg • Sodium: 17.9 mg • Zinc: 0.4mg • Each bar provides approximately ¼ fruit serving and 1 protein serving for children 1 to 3 years.

Strawberry-Banana Ice Cream

Bananas have a natural creaminess that makes a tasty frozen "dessert" when whipped up in a food processor or blender. The strawberries give this frozen banana ice cream an extra added boost of sweetness, but feel free to swap the strawberries for blueberries, mangoes, or whatever fresh or frozen fruit you have on hand. You will be truly amazed at how simple this is to make and how naturally delicious this tastes! | MAKES 1¼ TO 1⅔ CUPS

Pour the frozen bananas and strawberries into a blender or food processor. Blend until smooth and creamy. This will take a few minutes. Scrape down the sides and bottom of the bowl so all of the pieces of banana are blended. Blend in the optional heavy cream and peanut butter. Serve immediately.

Freeze for up to 1 month. When ready to serve, blend to restore the creamy consistency.

2 large ripe bananas, diced and frozen

½ cup frozen strawberries, or substitute with your child's favorite fruit

2 tablespoons heavy cream (optional)

2 tablespoons peanut butter (optional)

Note

To add calories, add 2 tablespoons of heavy cream for an additional 52 calories, 0.3 grams of protein, and 5.5 grams of fat per serving, or add 2 tablespoons peanut butter for an additional 100 calories, 3.5 grams of protein, and 8.0 grams of fat per serving.

Even though we like frozen bananas for their creaminess, to make this recipe even easier, feel free to experiment and blend your favorite bag of frozen fruit in a food processor to achieve similar results.

Prep time: 10 minutes

Excellent source for toddlers of fiber and vitamin C.

Good source for toddlers of protein, folate, and potassium.

Real Life Parenting

We like serving this "ice cream" to our toddlers not only for dessert but also as a quick breakfast with fresh fruit on top. Their eyes light up in disbelief when they learn they are having ice cream for breakfast!

NUTRIENTS PER SERVING: 1 serving: ¾ cup • Calories: 116.3 • Total Fat: 0.4 g • Saturated Fat: 0.1 g • Protein: 1.5 g • Carbohydrates: 30.2 g • Fiber: 3.8 g • Sugar: 15.9 g • Vitamin C: 23.8 mg • Calcium: 10.9 mg • Folate: 23.6 mcg • Iron: 0.5 mg • Potassium: 474.9 mg • Sodium: 1.2 mg • **Provides 1 fruit serving for children 1 to 3 years.**

Chapter Six

~~~~~~~~~~~~~~~~~~~~

Common Medical Conditions and Additional Resources

This chapter provides more detailed explanations of common medical conditions discussed throughout this book. It is divided into a gastrointestinal and nutritional section and an allergy section, with each part containing topics listed in alphabetical order for easy reference. We then discuss what a typical office visit to the dietitian, gastroenterologist, and allergist entails. We end with a list of useful websites and additional resources.

Common Gastrointestinal and Nutritional Conditions

This section will discuss the common gastrointestinal and nutritional conditions that may be faced in early infancy and childhood. We will review in more detail topics such as constipation, eosinophilic esophagitis, failure to thrive and feeding issues, gastroesophageal reflux, and gluten-related disorders.

Constipation

Constipation is a common condition that affects up to one-third of children. It is also a common reason for a visit to both the pediatrician and pediatric gastroenterologist. It is defined as a delay in or difficulty passing stool that lasts for two or more weeks. When discussing stool patterns, it is important to keep track of three things:

- **Change in frequency:** Every child is different, and therefore, there is no one "normal" stool frequency that all children must follow. Frequency varies based on the individual and age. Infants may not stool for many days (up to 10 to 14 days can be normal, especially in breastfeeding infants!) or may pass stool a few times a day, while children and adults stool every day to every other day.

- **Change in consistency:** Are the stools harder than normal? Do they look like a snake, soft-serve ice cream, or hard pellets? If it is soft (about the consistency of peanut butter), not painful for your child to pass, and your child is still acting normally and eating well, it is likely not constipation.

- **Ease of passage:** Does your child strain when stooling? Do you see blood? Any staining of underwear or pull-ups with stool? Straining is difficult to assess in infants since kids will usually make a "poopy" face while stooling. As your child gets older, they may have a dance or movements they make right before they stool or when they hold stool in. They may also be able to communicate whether they feel empty after they stool or whether they feel that there is more stool that they can't push out (which maybe a sign of constipation or stool retention).

Stool evacuation occurs through a combination of muscles and brain signals. The presence of a small amount of stool in the rectum activates stretch receptors, which leads to the relaxation of the internal anal sphincter. The stool then moves down the rectum to the external anal sphincter. Since infants do not have control of the external anal sphincter, stool will usually pass spontaneously. Infants will often stool with every feeding, due to the gastrocolic reflex. As children get older, they begin to control the external anal sphincter, so now in the presence of stool two things can happen: they can relax the external sphincter, squat, and stool; or they can tighten the external sphincter, and the stool migrates back up into the rectum. Stool that is withheld becomes harder, more difficult to pass, and as a result the colon can become stretched out. Some children who are very constipated may experience diarrhea or have stooling accidents as the softer stool leaks out around the harder stool in the stretched-out colon.

What is the most common cause of constipation?

Functional constipation is the most common reason for constipation. Functional means that there is no underlying medical or anatomic reason for constipation. In infants, rectal confusion is common. Infants will strain while stooling and this is normal due to poor coordination of pelvic floor muscles and how difficult it is to stool while lying down. Functional constipation can also be seen with toddlers, especially during potty training, when they withhold their stool. See chapter five for more on potty training.

Signs and Symptoms of Constipation

- Abdominal pain
- Butt pain
- Change in appetite
- Diarrhea (typically caused from overflow from a stretched-out colon)
- Encopresis and enuresis (stool and urine accidents, respectively)
- Rectal fissures
- Rectal prolapse (when rectal tissue slides out and protrudes through the anus). This finding may require further evaluation, so consult your pediatrician.

How is constipation diagnosed?

Your child's pediatrician will typically make the diagnosis based on a thorough history and physical exam. Your child's physician may perform a rectal exam to assess for rectal tone, stool impaction, and anal fissures. An abdominal X-ray, and occasionally an ultrasound, can help determine the extent of stool retention, as well as assess for whether dietary and/or medical treatment has been successful.

What diet modifications can help resolve constipation?

The first simple steps would include increasing fiber in the diet, drinking more water, exercising, and limiting constipating foods such as bananas and rice.

What medications can be used to treat constipation?

Some children will have improved stooling patterns quickly with basic diet changes; however, some children will need more chronic therapy. In general, the thought is that treatment will be needed for at least double the amount of time the symptoms have been present. For example, if your child has been constipated for three months, he/she will need to follow a treatment regimen for at least six months.

Medical therapy for chronic constipation can be divided into three parts:

1. **Evacuation:** Some children will require high-dose stool softeners to empty the colon. In most instances, this process may take a few days. Your child may need to wear pull-ups or at least have access to the potty. We recommend staying

at home during this time to limit stress and anxiety from frequent bowel movements. Possible medications include magnesium citrate, polyethylene glycol (PEG) 3350, pediatric fleet enemas, and glycerin suppositories.

2. **Maintain Evacuation:** Depending on the chronicity of your child's symptoms, your doctor may start with this phase and skip the evacuation phase. During this phase, medication doses are adjusted for a goal of one soft bowel movement on most days. This phase usually lasts for months and will be tailored according to your child's behavior and stooling pattern. Diet changes, such as adding fiber, may also be done at this time. Possible medications include PEG 3350, senna/Ex-Lax, and lactulose.

3. **Weaning Medications:** During this phase, your child's medications will be slowly decreased and hopefully completely weaned off. It is natural and normal, however, for a recurrence of symptoms to occur during changes in your child's life such as moving, birth of sibling, starting a new school, or going on vacation. Some children may require longer term therapy.

In general, it is important to start with diet changes. Suppositories should not be used regularly. Medications, although safe, may have side effects associated with them, and it is important to discuss the risks and benefits of using these medications with your physician.

Treatment of Constipation in Infants and Children

TREATMENT OPTIONS	TREATMENT OPTIONS FOR INFANTS	TREATMENT OPTIONS FOR CHILDREN
Diet changes	Add oatmeal or barley cereal Add prune/pear juice or pureed prunes/pears Decrease constipating foods including rice, bananas, and dairy (if on solid food)	Increase fruits and vegetables Increase water intake Decrease constipating foods and dairy
Medication	Lactulose Miralax/polyethylene glycol (PEG) 3350 Glycerin suppository	Magnesium citrate Magnesium Hydroxide Miralax/polyethylene glycol (PEG) 3350 Senna/Ex-Lax Lactulose Glycerin suppository Mineral Oil Fiber supplements Pediatric Fleet Enemas

What is fiber? How much fiber should my child eat?

Fiber is the part of plants that is indigestible, and it is an important part of a well-balanced diet. Fiber is a nutrient with many health benefits, such as maintaining healthy bowel habits.

There are no definitive fiber recommendations for children less than 1 year of age. However, it is recommended to slowly increase fiber from 6 to 12 months of life once complementary foods have been introduced into the diet. Fiber recommendations for children 1 to 3 years of age is 19 grams per day. If your child's diet is low on fiber, it's best to increase slowly to prevent any gastrointestinal distress, and also make sure your child is getting plenty of fluids. We recommend against the routine use of fiber supplements like fiber gummies, as they may contain added sugar, and don't have the extra health benefits of

Natural Sources of Fiber

FOOD	AMOUNT	FIBER (IN GRAMS)
Lentils, cooked	½ cup	7.8
Raspberries	½ cup	4
Whole-wheat spaghetti, cooked	½ cup	3.2
Broccoli, boiled	½ cup	2.6
Apple with skin	½ cup	2.2
Instant oatmeal, cooked	½ cup	2
Brown rice, cooked	½ cup	1.8

Fiber Supplements

NAME OF SUPPLEMENT	TYPE OF FIBER	AMOUNT OF FIBER
Benefiber (powder)	Wheat dextrin (soluble)	3 g per 2 teaspoons
Metamucil (powder)	Psyllium (insoluble)	3 g per teaspoon
L'il Critter Fiber Gummies	Polydextrose (soluble)	1.5 g per gummy

eating fruits and veggies. If your child has difficulty achieving fiber goals, talk to your pediatrician about adding a fiber supplement (see chart opposite).

What is the difference between soluble and insoluble fiber?

There are two types of fiber, soluble and insoluble. Soluble fiber is dissolvable in water, which helps to slow digestion and helps control blood sugar. Soluble fiber helps to lower cholesterol and helps prevent heart disease. Some good sources include oats, beans, nuts, seeds, and some fruits and vegetables including apples with skin and blueberries.

Insoluble fiber does not dissolve in water, thus it is able to speed the movement of food through the digestive tract and help prevent constipation. Good sources include whole wheat, brown rice, legumes, and vegetables such as broccoli.

Although, insoluble fiber is better for the treatment of constipation, we recommend concentrating on your child's overall intake of any fiber since typically foods will contain a bit of both soluble and insoluble fiber.

Eosinophilic Esophagitis

Eosinophilic esophagitis (or EoE) is a gastrointestinal condition in which the lining of the esophagus becomes inflamed due to an overabundance of white blood cells, called eosinophils. EoE is fairly rare (occurs approximately 1 in 2,000 people), affects children and adults, and is more common in boys than in girls.

What are the symptoms of eosinophilic esophagitis?

The symptoms can vary but can include reflux (heartburn), abdominal pain, recurrent or frequent vomiting, feeding and swallowing difficulties, poor appetite, poor weight gain and growth, pain with swallowing, or episodes of food getting stuck in the esophagus. It can present at any age and can be difficult to recognize or diagnose. The symptoms can wax and wane in severity, and can be difficult to distinguish from gastroesophageal reflux. It may be hard, especially for younger children, to describe or verbalize symptoms associated with esophageal discomfort.

How is eosinophilic esophagitis diagnosed?

The only way to confirm a diagnosis of EoE is by an upper endoscopy performed by a gastroenterologist. During an endoscopy, biopsy samples are taken from a few places along the esophagus. A pathologist then counts the number of eosinophils that are seen under the microscope from the sample. If there are more than 15 or 20 eosinophils in a very small area (in multiple areas of the esophagus), a diagnosis of EoE is suggested.

What is the treatment for eosinophilic esophagitis?

EoE can be treated with dietary or medical therapy. In some cases, EoE will go into remission on a "targeted elimination diet," or if one or a few foods are removed (most commonly milk or wheat). In other cases, a more restricted diet is necessary where the eight most common allergens are eliminated. In some more extreme cases, an elemental diet (limited to a hypoallergenic amino acid–based formula) is necessary. Treatment may also include antacids or topical steroids that treat the inflammation of the esophagus. Treatments, as well as the course of the disease, vary greatly from child to child.

Will my child outgrow EoE?

At this time, there is no known cure for EoE, and it is not known whether it will be a lifelong illness if it is diagnosed in childhood. Also, the way that this disease is managed may change over time, as we come to understand it better, and as new treatments are developed. The diagnosis and effective management of EoE really takes coordination and cooperation between the family and the child's doctors. In fact, children may need a whole team, including the pediatrician, gastroenterologist, allergist, and dietitian, to best care for their eosinophilic esophagitis.

For more information about eosinophilic esophagitis, please refer to the official website of the American Partnership for Eosinophilic Disorders, www.apfed.org.

Failure to Thrive and Feeding Problems

We discussed failure to thrive in chapter three. Please refer to that section for more details on this topic. Here we discuss ways to increase calories in the diet through naturally high-calorie foods as well as fortified nutritional supplements. In addition, in this section we will describe how to know if your child has a feeding problem and what evaluations are available for children with feeding issues.

How do I increase calories in my child's diet?

If you have been told your child is underweight or failure-to-thrive and needs additional calories, here are some suggestions on page 191 for foods and supplements that can add calories. These can be easily mixed into or sprinkled on top of your child's favorite meals. We recommend first adding high-calorie foods

High-Calorie Foods (per tablespoon)

FOODS	CALORIES	PROTEIN (GRAMS)	FAT (GRAMS)
Avocado	15	0.2	1.4
Butter	101	0.1	11.5
Chia seeds	60	3	4.5
Cheddar cheese	28.5	1.8	2.3
Cream cheese (whipped/brick)	35/50	1/0.9	3.5/5
Dried whole milk powder	40	2	2
Egg (per 1 large)	72	6	5
Feta cheese	28.5	1.8	2.3
Flaxseed meal	30	1.5	2.3
Heavy cream	52	0.3	5.5
Hummus	25	1.2	1.5
Parmesan cheese (varies depending on brand)	25–35	1.9–2.3	1.4–2.5
Peanut butter	100	3.5	8
Ricotta cheese	27	1.8	2
Sour cream	23.2	0.3	2.4
Vegetable oils (olive, canola, coconut, etc.)	113–126	0	14
Wheat germ	30	2	0.8

Source: ESHA The Food Processor Software.

Examples of High-Calorie Supplements

NAME	CALORIES	AVAILABLE FORMS	SOURCES OF CALORIES
Benecalorie	7.5 cal per mL	Liquid	Fat- and milk-based protein
Duocal	25 cal per scoop	Powder	Sugar and fat
Polycal	20 cal per scoop	Powder	Sugar only

Examples of Fortified Beverages (per 8-ounce serving)

NAME	CALORIES	PROTEIN (GRAMS)	FAT (GRAMS)
Pediasure	240	7	9
Boost Kid Essentials	240	7	9
Pediasmart Organic	240	7	9
Bright Beginnings Soy Pediatric Drink	240	7	12
Boost Breeze (juice supplement)	250	9	0
Pediasure 1.5	350	14	16

to your child's diet; however, your pediatrician may suggest some supplements as well (see chart above).

What are examples of nutritionally fortified beverages?

Nutritionally fortified beverages (see chart, above) are often recommended as a way to increase calories in children over 1 year who have a difficult time doing so with food alone. Children can drink these as a meal or snack, and usually the manufacturers provide suggestions on including these beverages in recipes. We do not recommend the use of these supplements without talking to your pediatrician.

How do I know if my child has a feeding problem?

Feeding problems are very common and many infants and young children exhibit food refusal and sensitivity, such as aversions to certain textured foods.

Some of these problems may be straightforward to manage, while other children may require more intensive evaluation and treatment.

Some questions to consider if you think your child is having feeding issues that may require further evaluation:

- Does your child take a disproportionately long time to eat? Mealtimes should not typically take more than thirty to forty-five minutes, and children who routinely require more time than this to complete a meal may warrant further evaluation.
- Are mealtimes particularly stressful for you or your child? Does your child have temper tantrums at meals, refuse food, spit up, or vomit in order to avoid eating?
- Is your child gaining weight appropriately? Children should gain weight steadily, especially in the first few years of life. If you feel that your child is not gaining weight, bring this to your pediatrician's attention.
- Does your child choke, gag, or vomit with meals? Your child may have gastroesophageal reflux disease (GERD) or an allergy. In addition, sometimes gagging and vomiting can occur in children who have sensory difficulties around food or as a food refusal tactic.
- Does your child have difficulty swallowing? For example, children with anatomic abnormalities may have difficulty swallowing solid foods. Some children have uncoordinated oral and pharyngeal phases of swallowing and are at an increased risk for aspiration of thin liquids; they are better able to swallow thicker textures.
- Does your child have sensitivity to certain food? While some food preferences are, of course, typical, some children have more significant sensory sensitivities to specific textures, colors, odors, tastes, or temperatures. They may gag easily when presented with specific types of foods, avoid getting their hands dirty, may not want to touch food, and avoid certain food textures. These differences can negatively impact feeding.

What types of evaluations and treatments are available for children with feeding problems?

If there are concerns about specific feeding problems, your child's doctor will likely recommend further evaluation and treatment. Some children will require specific diagnostic tests such as a video fluoroscopic or a modified barium swallow, especially if there are concerns about risk for aspiration or uncoordinated sucking and swallowing. These tests will monitor how your child handles and coordinates a swallow for thin to thickened liquids.

Gastroenterologists, developmental pediatricians, and pediatric feeding therapists have specific expertise in managing patients with feeding difficulties. Speech and language therapists perform oral feeding and swallowing evaluations and can provide feeding therapy. Occupational therapists evaluate and treat feeding issues that are related to problems around abnormal muscle tone, or sensory problems. If there are concerns around adequate weight gain and growth, a dietitian can assess and monitor your child's diet and nutritional needs.

Gastroesophageal Reflux and Gastroesophageal Reflux Disease

Gastroesophageal reflux (GER) is the movement of stomach contents into the esophagus, and possibly out through the mouth and nose. This usually means digested food or stomach secretions, including acid, will move into the esophagus. Gastroesophageal reflux is often referred to as spitting up. Though it may be messy and lead to a pile of laundry, it is often a normal process that occurs in many babies. When reflux is associated with symptoms or complications, or if it persists beyond infancy, it is considered a disease and is known as gastroesophageal reflux disease (GERD).

What are the causes of GER?

GER is very common in infants and children due to three main reasons:

1. The lower esophageal sphincter (LES) is shorter and does not elongate to the adult size until 2 years of age. This makes the muscle weaker so that food can easily bypass it and move back into the esophagus.

2. The diaphragm, a muscle located at the bottom of the rib cage, is located below the LES in infants, so it does not act as a protective barrier against acid reflux. In most adults, the muscle is located at the level of the LES, which adds to the antireflux barrier (see diagram page 43).

3. Normally, the LES will relax when we eat or drink to allow food or liquid to pass into the stomach and subsequently close. However, in children with GER, the muscle relaxation can happen randomly (before or after eating) and lasts longer than a typical relaxation, which can lead to regurgitation of stomach contents.

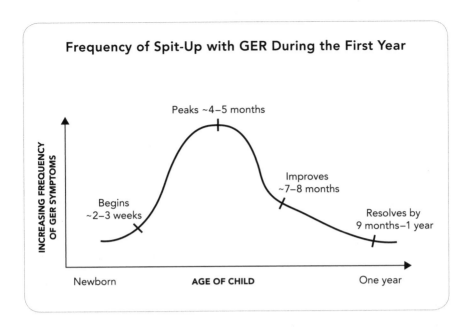

Frequency of Spit-Up with GER During the First Year

Peaks ~4–5 months

Improves ~7–8 months

Begins ~2–3 weeks

Resolves by 9 months–1 year

INCREASING FREQUENCY OF GER SYMPTOMS

Newborn   **AGE OF CHILD**   One year

How long does GER usually last?

The chart above shows spit-up frequency by age during infancy. Increased symptoms are noted up until 4 to 6 months of life and then begin to decrease.

Reflux in full-term infants usually starts at around 2 to 3 weeks of life, peaks at 4 to 5 months, and then will start getting better on its own. At 4 to 6 months of age, nearly 70 percent of infants will spit up at least once per day (possibly through the mouth and nose) and about 25 percent will spit up four or more times per day. By 7 to 8 months old, only 25 percent of babies will spit up at least once per day and less than 5 percent will spit up four or more times per day. Normal development, including improved head control and being able to sit up, as well as the introduction of solid food, will help improve GER. Children who are born prematurely or with decreased muscle tone, may have a slightly more prolonged course.

In older children, diet can play more of a role. Large meals and highly acidic or spicy meals, as well as carbonated or caffeinated beverages, can lead to increased GER symptoms. In addition, GER is more common in children who are overweight or obese.

What are the symptoms of GER and GERD?

It is often hard for parents (and doctors) to distinguish between GER and GERD because many of the symptoms overlap.

The following is a list of possible signs and symptoms that may be seen with either GER or GERD:

- Recurrent spit-up
- Mild feeding issues (for example occasional prolonged feeds or some feeds that are interrupted with the baby coming off the breast or bottle)
- Abdominal pain in older children
- Recurrent vomiting

These symptoms are more likely to be seen in GERD:

- Moderate to severe eating issues (for example arching of back or pain with feeding and most to all feedings interrupted or prolonged due to poor intake)
- Weight loss or poor weight gain
- Respiratory symptoms including wheezing and cough

Your child's physician will determine whether treatment is necessary based on persistence and intensity of these symptoms and your child's growth.

How will my doctor evaluate my child for GER and GERD?

In the majority of cases, your child will not need any diagnostic tests. Your doctor will take a history to review your child's symptoms and feeding patterns and will assess your child's growth by plotting his/her weight and height onto a growth chart. This information will help your physician determine whether your child is a "happy spitter" (when he/she spits up, they are not cranky and do not appear to be in pain) or has symptoms of GERD that may require medical therapy.

What are the available diagnostic tests for GER?

Sometimes diagnostic tests may be important to evaluate for *complications* from reflux and for other conditions that may be causing these symptoms to persist. The following is a list of these studies:

- **An upper gastrointestinal contrast study:** This test assesses your child's anatomy to make sure there is no blockage or obstruction that may be causing the vomiting. It requires your child to drink a liquid called contrast and the radiologist will take X-rays as the contrast moves down the esophagus, into the stomach, and into the first parts of the small intestines.
- **Upper endoscopy with biopsy:** An endoscope is a long tube with a camera at the tip. It allows for direct visualization of the upper

gastrointestinal tract, including the esophagus, stomach, and the first part of the small intestine. A gastroenterologist can take pictures and also superficial biopsies from the lining of the upper gastrointestinal tract to evaluate for causes of your child's symptoms, which can include assessing for inflammation, infection, allergy or celiac disease.

• **pH monitoring and impedance studies:** These tests can assess the extent and frequency of your child's reflux symptoms but is not done on a routine basis. A tube with sensors is placed through your child's nose into the esophagus. The sensors record the pH and impedance of the esophagus to detect acidic and non-acidic reflux, typically for twenty-four hours.

How is GER and GERD treated?

Dietary and behavioral modifications are typically the first-line treatments for gastroesophageal reflux and gastroesophageal reflux disease.

For infants, decreasing the volume of each feeding, feeding more frequently, frequent burping (usually after 1 to 2 ounces of milk or during a natural break from feeding), and being kept upright for approximately twenty to thirty minutes after feeding can be useful. Thickening bottles of expressed breast milk or formula with cereal may decrease the symptoms of reflux, but this should always be done under a doctor's advice.

For older kids, eating smaller meals, not lying down right after eating, and sleeping on their left side can be helpful. Limiting eating at least three hours prior to going to bed can also be beneficial. Diet changes include avoiding caffeine, carbonated beverages, chocolate, citrus fruits, tomato sauce, and spicy foods.

List of Foods to Avoid with GER or GERD

TYPES OF FOOD	EXAMPLES
Acidic foods	Tomatoes, ketchup, BBQ sauce Citrus fruits: lemon, lime, grapefruit, oranges, clementines, tangerines
Spicy foods	Chiles, hot peppers, hot sauce
Beverages and snacks	Seltzer water, soda Chocolate

What medications are available to treat GERD?

There are a variety of medications available for the treatment of acid reflux which decrease the amount of acid in the stomach. The majority of infants who have spit-up and reflux symptoms will either improve on their own or through dietary and behavioral changes. Treatment with medications may be indicated if your child has GERD and complications from reflux such as poor weight gain, respiratory symptoms and pain with vomiting. It is important to discuss whether your child should be started on these medications with your physician and possibly a pediatric gastroenterologist. Your physician will help you weigh the risks and benefits of these possible treatments.

The two more common medications used to treat reflux are histamine-2-receptor antagonists and proton pump inhibitors. These medications decrease the amount of stomach acid. Histamine-2-receptor antagonists such as ranitidine (Zantac), famotidine (Pepcid), and nizatidine (Axid), block one of the three pathways of acid production. They have been shown to relieve symptoms of acid reflux and aid in healing the lining of the esophagus. These medications are available in liquid formulations and require a prescription. They should ideally be given 30 minutes prior to eating for maximum effectiveness, which may be difficult since infants eat so frequently, and the medications are typically given two to three times a day.

Proton-pump inhibitors, such as esomeprazole (Nexium), lansoprazole (Prevacid), omeprazole (Prilosec), and pantoprazole (Protonix) block the release of acid into the stomach. There are a variety of brands and generic versions available. They come in dissolvable tablets, powdered form, and may be compounded into liquids. In older kids, capsules may be opened and the contents placed in applesauce. These medications should be given thirty minutes prior to eating and are usually given once to twice a day.

Occasionally, your physician may recommend an antacid such as Gaviscon, which helps neutralize gastric acid and can be taken before eating or as needed when symptoms develop. These medications contain magnesium and aluminum and there is no specific children's version available. You'll have to purchase the adult over-the-counter version and your doctor will recommend a dose based on your child's weight. Magnesium and aluminum may change the consistency of bowel movements.

Gluten-Related Disorders

In this section, we will review gluten-related disorders including celiac disease, wheat allergy, and non-celiac gluten sensitivity, and will discuss the signs and symptoms, diagnostic testing, and treatment options of each. We will also discuss the gluten-free diet and potential concerns. This section is designed to educate parents about these disorders so that if you think that gluten is the cause of any of your child's symptoms, you can discuss with your doctor if a diagnostic work-up is indicated and know whether a gluten-free diet is medically necessary.

What is gluten?

Gluten is a protein found in many different grains including rye, barley, and wheat.

Why is a gluten-free diet so popular?

Following a gluten-free diet has grown in popularity after many celebrities and medical professionals have described the potential benefits of eliminating gluten from the diet. From Lady Gaga and Miley Cyrus to the book *Wheat Belly* describing the potential and perceived negative effects of wheat, gluten has become associated with autoimmune diseases, neurologic disorders, and gastrointestinal symptoms. Research still needs to be done to better understand these possible associations.

The good news is that since the diet has increased in popularity, gluten-free foods are more available for those who need to follow it for medical reasons. Because there is an increase in demand, new gluten-free products are being introduced every year.

What is celiac disease?

Celiac disease is an immune-mediated disease where the exposure to gluten causes an inflammatory response in the lining of the intestines. This process causes the lining of the small intestines to become damaged (see diagram on page 202). Celiac disease occurs only in genetically susceptible individuals. This means you must carry at least one of the two genes associated with celiac disease: HLA-DQ2 or HLA-DQ8. However, carrying the gene is not enough. Approximately 30 to 40 percent of the population carries one of these genes, while only 1 in 133, or slightly less than 1 percent, actually develops celiac disease.

Can anything be done to prevent celiac disease?

There is not much known about what exactly causes some people who have one of the celiac genes to develop celiac while others do not. Recent studies have not demonstrated that breastfeeding can prevent celiac disease. Also, based on recent research, introduction of gluten at 6 months seems to be ideal, as delayed introduction beyond this age has not been found to prevent celiac disease. Infant barley or wheat cereals are good choices as the first gluten-containing food. Environmental factors may also play a role in those considered "at risk" (someone who carries one of the celiac genes), but more research is needed to better determine specific factors in the development of celiac disease.

Who is at higher risk for celiac disease?

Celiac is seen more commonly in children with type 1 diabetes, trisomy 21 (Down syndrome), immunoglobulin A deficiency, and a family history of celiac disease. Children in these high-risk groups should be routinely screened for celiac disease through blood testing. Repeat testing may be needed, since those at high risk for celiac disease can develop it at a later time.

What are symptoms of celiac disease?

There are many possible symptoms of celiac disease, including:

- Abdominal pain
- Abdominal bloating
- Short stature or slowed growth velocity
- Nausea or vomiting
- Lactose intolerance
- Constipation
- Poor weight gain or weight loss
- Diarrhea
- Iron deficiency that is not responsive to iron supplementation
- Rashes: the most common rash is dermatitis herpetiformis, which is a chronic itchy rash commonly found on the back of the neck, elbows, and knees.

In addition, some children may be asymptomatic and are diagnosed based on testing done for being "higher risk" as mentioned above.

What tests are used for diagnosis?

Serologic (blood) testing for celiac disease is the first step in the diagnosis of gluten-related disorders. Celiac testing varies from laboratory to laboratory and may include one or more of the following tests:

- **Total immunoglobulin A (total IgA):** This test is important. If normal, then the results of the celiac antibodies are accurate and can be believed. Otherwise, other antibodies may need to be checked.
- **Tissue transglutaminase IgA:** This is the test that is currently used routinely along with total IgA to screen someone for celiac disease. When this test is significantly elevated (more than ten times higher than the normal range), it is highly suggestive of celiac disease.
- **Deaminated gliadin IgG, endomysial IgA and tissue transglutaminase IgG:** These tests may also be elevated in children with celiac but are not checked routinely and are only checked in specific circumstances.
- **Celiac genetic markers, HLA-DQ2 and DQ8:** These tests are not routinely done since they can be expensive, but in certain situations may be helpful. They are done via a blood test or a cheek swab. A negative test is especially useful because this would then essentially eliminate the possibility of having or ever developing celiac. If positive, the tests do not mean much since 30 to 40 percent of the population carries at least one of the two celiac genes, and the majority of these children do not have nor will ever develop celiac disease.

What if the blood tests come back positive?

If the screening tests come back positive, please continue to include gluten in the diet until you review the blood tests with a gastroenterologist to determine the next steps. More diagnostic testing, including additional blood work and an upper endoscopy, may be indicated.

During the endoscopy, which requires sedation, biopsies will be taken in the duodenum (the first part of the small intestine). The samples will be looked at under a microscope to visualize the intestines. When you look under the microscope at the intestines, you can see fingerlike regions called villi, which is the area of the intestines where absorption occurs. In celiac disease, the villi can be irritated, shortened, or lost. The villi and intestines will usually return to normal after being on a gluten-free diet.

Intestinal Changes with Celiac Disease

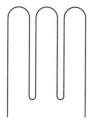 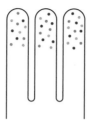 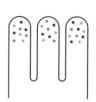

Normal villi without inflammation

Inflammation at tips of villi

Villous blunting or shortening

Villous atrophy or loss of villi

This image compares the intestinal villi, as seen under a microscope, in a person without celiac disease (left) to a person with celiac disease (all other images).

What is wheat allergy?

Wheat allergy is an IgE immune-mediated response that consistently and repeatedly occurs with the ingestion of wheat. It may lead to gastrointestinal symptoms (diarrhea, vomiting, abdominal pain), a rash, or any other allergic symptoms (see page 206). Screening for wheat allergy is important, especially if screening tests for celiac are negative.

What is gluten sensitivity?

Gluten sensitivity (also referred to as non-celiac gluten sensitivity) is not a well-defined entity and some physicians question the validity of the diagnosis. Other physicians feel that gluten sensitivity is only due to a wheat intolerance and not other gluten-containing grains such as rye and barley. The term is used to diagnose individuals with symptoms similar to celiac disease, whose diagnostic testing for celiac disease and wheat allergy are negative.

The prevalence of gluten sensitivity is not fully understood. While some studies have estimated that 8 percent or more of the population may have gluten sensitivity, more recently it appears that the actual numbers may be lower, particularly in children, with prevalence estimated to be much less than that of celiac disease. More studies are needed to better define the exact criteria for diagnosis of nongluten celiac sensitivity.

Cross-Contamination

When eating outside of the home, certain foods may contain gluten either as an ingredient or through cross-contamination that can occur when a gluten-free food comes in contact with a gluten-containing product. It is important to be smart when eating out so if the ingredients cannot be verified, eat something you know will be safe.

Examples of foods that may contain or be cross-contaminated with gluten:

- Fried foods (restaurants do not always have a separate fryer so fried food can be easily cross-contaminated)
- Broths from Chinese restaurants
- Pizza
- Sandwich shops
- California rolls (imitation crab has gluten!) from sushi restaurants
- Communion wafers
- Candy
- Herbal teas
- Drink mixes
- Soy sauce

Examples of other common products that may contain gluten:

- Play-Doh
- Shampoo and conditioner
- Toothpaste
- Mouthwash
- Certain medications: speak to your physician, pharmacist, and check www.glutenfreedrugs.com to verify that medications are truly gluten-free.

What tests are done for gluten sensitivity and wheat allergy?

There are tests available for gluten sensitivity, but they are expensive, unreliable, typically not covered by insurance, and not FDA regulated. Most importantly, these tests are not helpful in diagnosing gluten sensitivity. Therefore, there are no standardized tests that physicians use for gluten sensitivity and a diagnosis is based on symptoms. For wheat allergy, a pediatrician or allergist will decide whether skin prick testing or serum RAST testing in indicated based on your child's symptoms.

What treatment options are available?

A gluten-free diet is the only currently available treatment for celiac disease and gluten-related disorders. It can be difficult to follow, especially when eating at school, friends' parties, or restaurants. There are many gluten-free foods available now and with the new 2014 FDA labeling regulations for gluten-free products (if a food label claims that a product is gluten-free, it must contain less than 20 parts per million of gluten), hopefully the risk of cross-contamination will decrease (see sidebar on page 203).

Gluten-free foods tend to be high in sugar and fat and not as fortified in vitamins and minerals, especially in calcium, B vitamins, and vitamin D. Studies in children have demonstrated that the majority of kids gain weight on a gluten-free diet even if they were at an appropriate weight prior to the diagnosis. It is recommended that most kids start on a multivitamin with iron at the time of diagnosis. It is also recommended to consume naturally gluten-free foods.

What are gluten-free grains and other foods my child can eat?

It is important when following a gluten-free diet to choose foods that are safe for your child to eat. Though eating gluten-free may seem hard at first, there are many naturally gluten-free foods (fruits, vegetables, meats, poultry, fish, and eggs) and gluten-free grains available to eat (see chart opposite).

Can I eat oats?

Oats are gluten-free, though there may be some cross-contamination since they are grown near gluten-containing grains. Most children with celiac disease and gluten-related disorders tolerate oats quite well. However, we recommend eating oats or oat products that are labeled gluten-free and limiting the daily intake of gluten-free dry oats to about 50 grams per day, which is the equivalent of 1/2 cup dry rolled oats or granola a day.

Allergic Conditions and Treatments

This section will discuss food allergies, cow's milk protein allergy, and food protein–induced enterocolitis syndrome. Please see pages 224 and 225 "Tips for Avoiding Your Allergen" as well as www.foodallergy.org/faap for the Food Allergy an Anaphylaxis Emergency Care Plan.

GRAINS CONTAINING GLUTEN	WHEAT DERIVATIVES	GLUTEN-FREE GRAINS	NATURALLY GLUTEN-FREE FOODS
• Barley	• Bulgur	• Amaranth	• Beans and legumes
• Brewer's yeast	• Couscous	• Arrowroot	• Dairy
• Malt	• Durum	• Buckwheat	• Eggs
• Rye	• Einkorn	• Corn	• Fish
• Triticale	• Emmer	• Flax	• Fruit
• Wheat	• Farina	• Millet	• Meat and poultry
	• Farro	• Montina	• Nuts
	• Graham	• Oats*	• Vegetables
	• Matzo	• Quinoa	
	• Semolina	• Rice	
	• Spelt	• Sorghum	
	• Wheat berries	• Tapioca	
	• Wheat starch	• Teff	

*Gluten-free oats may be consumed in limited amounts (see page 204).

Food Allergies

Food allergies (IgE-mediated or classical food allergies) affect one in thirteen children, and have become more prevalent in the past two decades. Many food allergies first present during infancy and early childhood. A food allergy (or any allergic reaction) occurs when the immune system recognizes a typically harmless protein as a threat. The immune system responds by "attacking" and trying to quickly rid the body of the protein, but in the process provokes an "allergic reaction." For example, the immune response that is activated is responsible for many symptoms, such as itching, hives, swelling, sneezing, wheezing, coughing, difficulty breathing, abdominal pain, vomiting, and even low blood pressure and poor circulation. Sometimes this allergic response is a severe anaphylactic reaction.

What causes an allergy?

Specific IgE antibodies are partly responsible for the allergic response, and this is the reason that this type of food allergy is called IgE-mediated food allergy. This type of food allergy is very different from a food intolerance or food sensitivity; although sometimes the term "allergy" is incorrectly used to refer to other responses that children have to foods.

An allergic reaction may happen when feeding a baby a new food, and is most often is seen with only a few foods (milk, eggs, soy, wheat, peanuts, tree nuts, sesame, fish, and shellfish). This list of foods is not exclusive, and an allergy can occur to almost any food. Although less common, an allergy can occur to a food that has already been tried a few times without any reaction. However, in the vast majority of cases, an allergic reaction does not develop to a food that has already been a regular or consistent part of a child's diet.

What are symptoms of an allergic response?

Allergic reactions are not all the same. Most allergic reactions start within minutes to an hour after eating a causative food, although reactions that are delayed several hours are possible. The spectrum of allergic reactions ranges from very mild skin reactions or transient gastrointestinal discomfort to severe anaphylaxis. Minor allergic reactions resolve spontaneously and quickly, while more serious allergic reactions are true emergencies and require prompt treatment and medical attention. An allergic reaction can also progress to involve more symptoms over time. In some cases, a patient may even develop a "biphasic reaction" or a second phase of anaphylaxis several hours after recovering from the initial reaction. The following are symptoms that can be seen during an allergic reaction:

Lung: Short of breath, wheezing, repetitive cough

Heart: Pale, blue, faint, weak pulse, dizzy

Throat: Tight, hoarse, trouble breathing or swallowing

Mouth: Significant swelling of the tongue or lips (mild version: itchy mouth)

Skin: Many hives, widespread redness (mild version: a few hives, mild itch)

Gut: Repetitive vomiting, severe diarrhea (mild version: slight nausea or discomfort)

What should I do if my child has a food allergy?

If you know that your child has a food allergy, it is very important that you speak with your pediatrician or allergist, and that you educate yourself regarding anaphylaxis. You should review the signs and symptoms of anaphylaxis, have an updated and personalized emergency treatment plan (www.foodallergy.org/faap), have a nonexpired epinephrine autoinjector always available (remember to keep one at your child's school or daycare as well as at home), and make sure that you (and any caregivers for your child) know how and when to use epinephrine. It is also important to practice with the epinephrine training devices every three months to ensure that you always know how to use them properly. Please see epinephrine dosing on page 210 for more information.

Will my child's food allergies resolve?

Many food allergies that appear in infancy do resolve during childhood. Most children who have allergies to milk, egg, soy, and wheat will eventually outgrow these food allergies, often in early childhood, before school-age. Infants and children who can tolerate milk and eggs in baked or well-heated forms tend to outgrow their milk and egg allergies even more rapidly. Allergies to peanuts, tree nuts, and seafood are less likely to be outgrown, but can be transient or resolve in some cases. Children who have known food allergies should be followed regularly by a pediatrician or an allergist, as allergy testing over time (via skin prick tests and IgE levels) can indicate when and if food allergies are likely to resolve. If your baby or child has been diagnosed with a food allergy, it is important not to try refeeding the allergenic food at home without first discussing this with your pediatrician or allergist. In many cases, an allergist will suggest a doctor-supervised feeding test (or an "oral food challenge") to confirm in a safe, controlled, medical office setting whether a food allergy has been outgrown.

An excellent source and starting point for information about food allergies is the Food Allergy Research and Education (FARE) website, www.foodallergy.org.

Cow's Milk Protein Allergy or Allergic Protocolitis

Cow's milk–induced proctocolitis (allergic proctocolitis) is a relatively benign and fairly common milk intolerance that can present in the first few weeks or months of a baby's life. It most commonly occurs in breast-fed infants, but can develop in formula-fed babies as well.

What are the symptoms of allergic proctocolitis? How is it diagnosed?

Babies with allergic proctocolitis present with visible blood in their stool (sometimes flecks or streaks), and the stool is often loose and mucousy. Sometimes parents will perceive that their baby is also uncomfortable or more colicky. Rarely, children may not be gaining weight appropriately, but more often the baby is not bothered at all, and will otherwise eat, sleep, and behave normally. If your pediatrician thinks your baby has allergic proctocolitis they might refer you to a gastroenterologist. A stool sample may be examined by the gastroenterologist and assessed for blood and allergic inflammatory cells.

What is the treatment for allergic proctocolitis?

Treatment of allergic proctocolitis generally entails completely removing cow's milk from the breastfeeding mother's diet, or a switch from a milk-based infant formula to an extensively hydrolyzed protein or amino acid–based infant formula (see chapter one for details on these formula options). Thirty to fifty percent of babies who have this sensitivity to milk will also react similarly to soy, so soy formula is not a recommended alternative, and a breastfeeding mother will also be advised to remove soy from her own diet. Rarely, other food proteins (egg, corn, and some grains) may be causing the symptoms and need to be removed from a breastfeeding mom's diet as well. Once milk and soy are removed from the mother's diet, and, if applicable, from the baby's diet, the allergic proctocolitis symptoms should resolve in three to five days, meaning that when you look at your baby's stool, blood should no longer be seen. However, blood may still be seen microscopically for weeks. If the symptoms do not resolve when milk and soy are strictly avoided, further evaluation may be necessary. The majority of babies with allergic proctocolitis outgrow this sensitivity between 9 to 12 months of life, without any long-term health effects. Some children do, however, have a more persistent form of allergic proctocolitis that requires avoidance of milk and soy, usually until 18 months to 2 years of age. See page 37 for more details on allergic proctocolitis.

Food Protein–Induced Enterocolitis Syndrome

Food protein-induced enterocolitis syndrome (FPIES) is a non-IgE mediated response to food that usually presents in young infants with episodes of repetitive severe vomiting, followed by diarrhea, starting several hours after the baby ingests the causative food. Diarrhea may persist for several hours or more after the vomiting stops. FPIES episodes can be significant enough to lead to dehydration, especially in young infants, and intravenous fluid hydration may be needed. The good news is that children usually outgrow FPIES by 3 to 5 years of age and though the symptoms of vomiting and diarrhea can be severe, the reaction is not associated with anaphylaxis (see page 50 for more information).

When does FPIES typically present?

FPIES usually presents when solid foods are introduced into a baby's diet (around 4 to 6 months of age) and is mostly commonly triggered by rice, wheat, oat, sweet potato, or poultry, but can happen with other foods as well. FPIES can also happen earlier, in the first months of life, with exposure to milk or soy formulas, but very rarely occurs in babies who are exclusively breastfeeding before they are exposed to solid foods. An FPIES reaction can also occur upon trying a food for the third or fourth time. Generally, a child does not have more than one to three foods that trigger FPIES reactions.

How is FPIES diagnosed? What is the treatment for FPIES?

A child with a suspected FPIES reaction should be evaluated by an allergist or gastroenterologist who is familiar with this condition. There is no laboratory or skin test that can confirm this form of delayed allergy, however, and a diagnosis of FPIES is generally based on a history of characteristic symptoms and a physical exam. Parents need to be instructed on careful avoidance of the causative food, and need to know how to manage or seek help if an FPIES reaction does occur. At this point, there is no cure for FPIES. We still have a lot to learn about FPIES and there is active research into this unusual form of food reaction.

Benadryl Dosing Chart

WEIGHT	CHILDREN'S LIQUID SUSPENSION (12.5 MG/5 ML)
11 lb to 16 lb, 7 oz	½ tsp or 2½ ml
16 lb, 8 oz to 21 lb, 15 oz	¾ tsp or 3¾ ml
22 lb to 26 lb, 7 oz	1 tsp or 5 ml
27 lb, 8 oz to 32 lb, 15 oz	1¼ tsp or 6¼ ml
33 lb to 37 lb, 7 oz	1½ tsp or 7½ ml
38 lb, 8 oz to 43 lb, 15 oz	1¾ tsp or 8¾ ml
44 lb to 54 lb, 15 oz	2 tsp or 10 ml
55 lb to 65 lb, 15 oz	2½ tsp
66 lb to 76 lb, 15 oz	3 tsp
77 lb to 87 lb, 5 oz	3½ tsp
88 lb +	4 tsp

Courtesy of Pediatric Associate of NYC, PC.

For more information and resources about FPIES, you may wish to visit the website for the International FPIES Association at www.fpies.org.

Diphenhydramine Dosing (Brand Name: Benadryl)

Benadryl is an antihistamine, so it can be used for allergic reactions, allergies, and for cough and cold symptoms. It can be given every six hours, as needed. Benadryl and generic forms of diphenhydramine come in a liquid suspension for children (see chart on page 209 for dosing).

Epinephrine Dosing

Self-injectable epinephrine devices are syringes prefilled with epinephrine (adrenalin) that are connected to a spring-activated needle mechanism that allows for very rapid injection of epinephrine to the mid/outer thigh. In the United States, epinephrine is currently available as a prescription in only two premeasured dose options: 0.15mg and 0.3mg. Epinephrine autoinjector prescriptions are given based on weight, but there is not as much flexibility as we would like in terms of the available devices.

- For a child less than 22 pounds (10 kg), there is no appropriately dosed epinephrine autoinjector available. If your child falls into this category, you will need to discuss with your doctor whether it is appropriate to have a 0.15 milligrams dose autoinjector.
- For children 22 to 33 pounds (10 kg to 15 kg), the 0.15 milligrams epinephrine device is usually prescribed, even though the amount of medicine may be more than what is needed based on your child's weight. However, the benefit of using epinephrine in a timely manner for a severe reaction far outweighs this risk.
- For children 33 pounds to 66 pounds (15 kg to 30 kg), the 0.15 mg (0.15 ml, 1:2000) epinephrine device is appropriate.
- For any individual (child or adult) 66 pounds (30 kg) and above, the 0.3 mg (0.3 ml, 1:1000) epinephrine device is appropriate.

These dosing parameters are what are currently recommended. Please review with your doctor, however, for your child's recommended dose. This is meant to be a guide and not as a substitute for your doctor's advice.

It is recommended that any person who has been prescribed an epinephrine autoinjector device, always have access to two devices, as sometimes a second dose is needed to treat an anaphylactic reaction. This is why the major manufacturers of epinephrine devices provide these as "two-sets" or "twin-packs" (with a trainer that contains no medication). The two devices should always be kept together. Also, always make sure you know which one is the trainer and which one is the actual device with medication—a trainer will not treat an allergic reaction.

Epinephrine has an expiration date and specific storage instructions. Make sure you replace your devices, that you always have unexpired medication, and that you store them at the correct temperature. Review the package insert for more about the storage instructions.

Epipen® (Epinephrine) Auto-Injector Directions
1. Remove the EpiPen Auto-Injector from the plastic carrying case.
2. Pull off the blue safety release cap.
3. Swing and firmly push orange tip against mid-outer thigh.
4. Hold for approximately 10 seconds.
5. Remove and massage the area for 10 seconds.

Visiting a Specialist

In this section we will explain when a referral to a dietitian, gastroenterologist, and allergist may be necessary. We also describe what a typical visit to each of these specialists would entail.

Dietitian

Registered dietitians are food and nutrition experts. They help give practical dietary advice based on scientific evidence. Anyone can legally call themselves a nutritionist (including the employee at your local health food store), but only a registered dietitian has completed education and training established by the Academy of Nutrition and Dietetics.

Your pediatrician may advise that your child see a dietitian for assistance with diet and lifestyle planning for conditions such as:

- Overweight and obesity
- Failure to thrive and underweight
- Food allergies or intolerances
- Excessive picky eating
- Vegetarian or other special diets

What does a typical visit entail?

During a typical visit with a dietitian, your child will be weighed and measured. The dietitian may ask about your child's health history, growth patterns, family medical history, medications and supplements, allergies, and eating habits, and will usually obtain a detailed twenty-four-hour diet recall. During a twenty-four-hour diet recall, your dietitian will ask you to remember everything your child ate and drank in the twenty-four hours prior to the visit. Your dietitian may show you food models or photos to help you gauge the portion sizes your child ate. Your dietitian will assess all the given information, and with your assistance and feedback, come up with a personally tailored nutritional plan and goals for your child. Follow-up visits are often necessary to monitor progress and adjust the plan based on your child's age or change in condition.

What is three-day calorie count?

Usually, a detailed twenty-four-hour diet recall during a visit can give a dietitian enough information to create an appropriate plan; however, sometimes more detailed information is needed, and therefore your dietitian or pediatrician may ask for a three-day food record or calorie count. You will be asked to write down everything your child eats and drinks for three days. These are most useful when done over three consecutive days, and ideally should include one weekend day. You will be asked to provide details about serving sizes, food preparation method, and the time food was consumed. This method allows a dietitian to determine a more reliable estimate of nutrient consumption.

Pediatric Gastroenterologist

A pediatric gastroenterologist is a pediatrician with specialized training in diseases involving the gastrointestinal tract (which includes the esophagus, stomach, small and large intestines) and the liver. Common reasons why your pediatrician may refer your child to see a pediatric gastroenterologist include:

- Poor weight gain
- Vomiting
- Chronic constipation
- Diarrhea
- Bloody stools
- Gastroesophageal reflux disease
- Feeding problems

- Food allergies affecting the gastrointestinal tract, such as cow's milk protein–induced proctocolitis and eosinophilic (allergic) esophagitis
- Chronic abdominal pain
- Celiac disease
- Inflammatory bowel disease

What should I expect from the visit?

During the first visit, the gastroenterologist will review the reason for your visit and ask you about your child's past medical and birth history. He/she will review any medical records and any testing that may have already been done. Your doctor may recommend blood, stool, or radiologic studies, including an abdominal ultrasound or an abdominal X-ray. To further understand your child's issues, a pediatric gastroenterologist may recommend additional testing such as an upper endoscopy and/or colonoscopy, which are special tests that require sedation and allow your gastroenterologist to see the lining of the gastrointestinal tract.

Endoscopy and Colonoscopy

During an upper endoscopy, an endoscope (or long tube with a camera at the tip) is passed through your child's mouth and into the esophagus, stomach, and small intestine. During a colonoscopy, the colonoscope is passed through the anus and then into and around the colon. The doctor can take pictures during these tests, but more importantly can take small biopsies in each of these areas. These biopsies can be helpful to diagnose the cause of your child's symptoms.

Allergist

An allergist (or immunologist) is a doctor who has specialized training in disorders of the immune system. They are specially equipped to evaluate and manage many types of allergies, including allergies to foods, environmental allergens (like pets and mold), vaccines, medications, and insect stings. They manage conditions that may be a manifestation of or caused by allergies, including asthma, hay fever, eczema and hives. Often, an allergic person may see an allergy specialist for several conditions and, since allergies run in families, many allergists take care of several people in the same family. In addition, an allergist may evaluate children who have recurrent infections (more than normal colds during the winter months) to help determine whether the immune system is functioning properly or if a child might be immune deficient. Allergists also have a good understanding of autoimmune diseases and tend to work closely with other specialists like dermatologists, gastroenterologists, and pulmonologists, who may coordinate care of certain medical problems.

Your pediatrician knows very well when an allergy consultation would be helpful or is needed, and may be able to steer you away from unnecessary testing when it is not needed—don't be afraid to ask! As this book is focused on infant and toddler feeding, here are some of the common reasons for recommending a child be evaluated for food allergies:

- A baby or child who has had immediate allergic symptoms (for instance hives, itching, generalized pink rash, lip swelling, vomiting, diarrhea, wheezing, coughing, or hoarse voice) within minutes to hours after eating a new or recently introduced food, especially if it is one of the top nine allergens (milk, eggs, soy, wheat, fish, shellfish, peanuts, tree nuts, or sesame).
- An infant who has had repetitive vomiting episodes after eating a specific food.
- A child who has moderate to severe eczema that is persistent over several months and does not respond adequately to moisturizing skin care and low potency topical steroids.
- An infant or child with a diagnosis of (or where there is a suspicion of) eosinophilic gastrointestinal disease (including eosinophilic esophagitis) and for some cases of allergic proctocolitis.
- In some instances, for a child with a strong first-degree family history of food allergies (in a parent or older sibling), or who is at high risk for developing food allergies.

What does a typical allergy visit entail?

Overall, there is no typical allergy visit, as every patient and problem is unique. Allergists will gear evaluation, forms of testing, and follow-up recommendations to each patient based on medical history and physical exam. For food allergies, allergists can perform two types of tests: skin prick test (sometimes called a "scratch test") or measurement of specific food IgE levels in the blood (this involves obtaining a blood sample). Both of these forms of allergy testing essentially measure the same thing, which is the allergic antibody response to a specific protein or allergen.

Skin prick testing is a very good way to test for food allergies. It is safe, not painful (but may be itchy), and can provide important information in less than fifteen minutes! Skin prick testing involves the placement of a small drop of a commercially made allergenic food extract on the skin (on the back or forearm), and pricking or scratching the skin under the drop with a special sterile skin prick device. Generally, several foods or panels of foods are placed at one time, although most allergists will limit the number of tests in a small child or infant. After a period of about ten minutes, the skin test sites are observed for the appearance of small wheals (or hives), and these positive tests are measured and recorded. An allergen that does not produce a wheal is considered a negative test. A positive skin test indicates the presence of food-specific IgE, but does not tell you for sure if a child is allergic to a specific food. False positive tests are possible (the test may be positive, but your child may not actually be allergic to the food).

An allergist (or your pediatrician) may also draw blood to determine specific IgE levels to different foods. There may be reasons to do blood tests instead of skin tests—for instance, if your child is on an antihistamine medication that cannot be stopped or if he/she has very significant eczema covering most of his/her skin. Many allergists may initially do both skin testing and serum IgE testing as part of their evaluation of food allergies or will do these tests on a yearly basis. Interpreting the results requires a fair amount of experience and knowledge. Of course, sometimes after listening to a patient history, an allergist may decide that testing is not necessary—it all depends!

Many children who have food allergies will outgrow some or all of their allergies. Sometimes, however, the above allergy tests are not adequate for determining whether it is safe to start having certain foods at home. In these cases, an allergist will suggest a supervised "oral food challenge." The oral food challenge allows for the food to be tried gradually, and in a safe, controlled doctor's office setting, where expertise and equipment for treating an allergic reaction are readily available. The oral food challenge generally involves having a child eat a food in small increments spaced over an hour, followed by several hours of observation after the food is consumed. If there is no reaction, then an oral food challenge is considered negative and the child can continue to eat the food at home. A positive oral challenge is one in which there is an observed allergic reaction (which would be treated by the allergist in the office), and proves that there is an allergy to a specific food, and that it will still need to be avoided at home.

Table of Major Nutrients, Their Function, and Recommended Intake

Nutrient	Function	Food Source
Fat	Concentrated energy source. Trans fats, saturated fats, and cholesterol are not as healthy as polyunsaturated or monounsaturated or "good" fats.	Breast milk and formula, butter, cream, oils, protein-rich foods like non lean meats and fish, full fat dairy, eggs, nuts and seeds
Protein	Energy source	Breast milk and formula, meats, poultry, fish, legumes such as beans and peas, tofu, eggs, nuts/seeds, dairy including cheese and yogurt
Carbohydrates	Energy source	Breast milk and formula, fruits and veggies, whole grains such as breads and cereals, potatoes, corn
Fiber	Fiber is the part of plants that is indigestible. It has many health benefits, such as maintaining healthy bowel habits and decreasing the risk of coronary artery disease.	Beans (navy, kidney, black, lima, white), lentils, many fruits and vegetables including artichokes, broccoli, apples with skin on
Vitamin A	Fat-soluble vitamin needed for normal immune function, vision, reproduction, cell growth, and wound healing.	Breast milk and formula, egg yolks, dark green veggies, yellow veggies, orange fruits, pistachios, ricotta cheese
Vitamin B_{12}	Involved in red blood cell formation.	Breast milk, infant formula, fortified breakfast cereals, salmon, beef, ham, egg, poultry
Vitamin C	Involved in wound healing, keeps teeth healthy.	Breast milk and formula, fruits (citrus fruits, strawberries, cantaloupe), vegetables (potatoes, broccoli, Brussels sprouts, cauliflower)
Vitamin D	Fat-soluble vitamin needed for bone health.	Infant formula, fatty fish like salmon, fortified orange juice, fortified milk, fortified yogurt, margarine, sardines, beef liver, eggs, fortified cereals, sunlight
Vitamin E	Antioxidant	Breast milk, formula, wheat germ, vegetable oils, liver, egg yolks, sunflower seeds, almonds, peanut butter, spinach, broccoli, mango, tomato

Recommended Daily Intake

0–6 months*	7–12 months	1–3 years	During Lactaction (>18 years)
31 g	30 g*	30–40% of diet	20–35% of diet
9.1 g	11 g	13 g	71 g
60 g	95 g*	130 g*	210 g*
Increase gradually over the course of 1 year of age		19 g	29g
400 mcg	500 mcg*	300 mcg	1300 mcg
0.4 mcg	0.5 mcg	0.9 mcg	2.8 mcg
40 mg	50 mg	15 mg	120 mg
400 IU	400 IU	600 IU	600 IU
4 mg	5 mg*	6 mg	19 mg

Table continues on pp. 218–219

Table continues from pp. 216–217

Table of Major Nutrients, Their Function, and Recommended Intake

Nutrient	Function	Food Source
Vitamin K	Aids in forming blood clots and stopping bleeding.	Infant formula, vegetable oils, liver, green leafy vegetables
Calcium	Important for muscle and nerve function, bone and teeth health, and blood clotting.	Breast milk and formula, yogurt, milk, cheese, fortified orange juice, tofu, salmon, kale, sardines
Folate	Important during pregnancy to prevent spinal cord defects. Also involved in red blood cell maturation.	Breast milk and formula, cooked spinach, asparagus, black-eyed peas, fortified and enriched grain products, oranges, beef, avocado
Iron	Important for oxygen transport.	Breast milk and formula, fortified breakfast cereals, oysters, white beans, chicken, meat, lentils, spinach, tofu, kidney beans, cashews
Omega-3 Fatty Acids	Plays a role in neurological development and growth and cardiac health.	Oils (soybean, canola, flax seed and fish), fatty fish, small amounts in meat and eggs
Potassium	Maintains cell function, and blood pressure, and important in bone and kidney health.	Fruits, vegetables, dairy foods, meats, nuts
Sodium	Maintains water balance in the body and regulates blood volume.	Table salt; foods with added salt such as soups, salted meats, salted nuts, and other processed foods
Zinc	Mineral that plays a role in immune function and protein synthesis.	Breast milk and formula, oysters, beef, crab, fortified breakfast cereal, lobster, pork chop, baked beans, chicken, yogurt, almonds, egg yolk.

Adapted from NIH, Pediatric Nutrition Handbook, *6th Edition, and from the USDA WIC Program*

Recommended Daily Intake

Recommended Dietary Allowances (RDAs) are the average daily dietary intake levels sufficient to meet the nutrient requirements of nearly all (97–98 percent) healthy individuals in a group. If there is not sufficient scientific evidence to establish an RDA, an Adequate Intake (AI) is usually developed. AIs are the dietary intake levels that are assumed to cover the needs of individuals in the group, but there may *(continues on page 219)*

Recommended Daily Intake

0–6 months*	7–12 months	1–3 years	During Lactaction (>18 years)
2.0 mcg	2.5 mcg*	30 mcg*	90 mcg*
200 mg	260 mg*	700 mg	1000 mg
65 mcg	80 mcg*	150 mcg	500 mcg
0.27 mg	11 mg	7 mg	9 mg
0.5 g	0.5 g*	0.7 g*	1.3 g*
400 mg	700 mg*	3000 mg*	5100 mg*
120 mg	370 mg*	1000 mg*	1500 mg*
2 mg	3 mg	3 mg	12 mg

be a lack of data or uncertainty in the data that prevents being able to specify with confidence the percentage of individuals covered by this intake. In the chart above, we use AI for 0–6 months and anywhere you see an asterisk (*) after the value. (Source: Texas Children's Hospital Pediatric Reference Guide, and http://ods.od.nih.gov/Health_Information/Dietary_Reference_Intakes.aspx)

Monitoring Your Child's Growth

These are growth charts for boys and girls from birth to 36 months from the
Centers for Disease Control and Prevention, an American government agency.

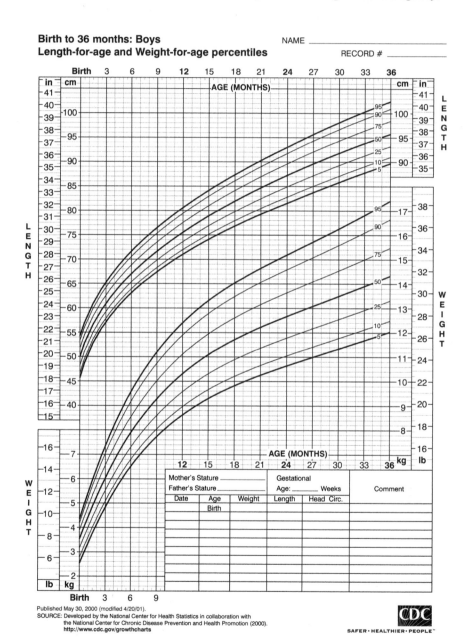

Birth to 36 months: Boys
Length-for-age and Weight-for-age percentiles

NAME _____

RECORD # _____

Published May 30, 2000 (modified 4/20/01).
SOURCE: Developed by the National Center for Health Statistics in collaboration with
the National Center for Chronic Disease Prevention and Health Promotion (2000).
http://www.cdc.gov/growthcharts

CDC
SAFER · HEALTHIER · PEOPLE™

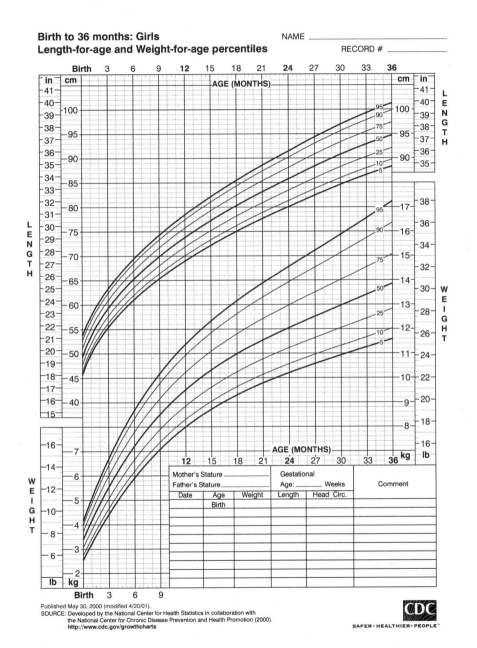

Birth to 36 months: Girls
Length-for-age and Weight-for-age percentiles

NAME _____

RECORD # _____

Published May 30, 2000 (modified 4/20/01).
SOURCE: Developed by the National Center for Health Statistics in collaboration with
the National Center for Chronic Disease Prevention and Health Promotion (2000).
http://www.cdc.gov/growthcharts

These are growth charts for boys and girls from birth to 24 months from the World Health Organization, a United Nations agency.

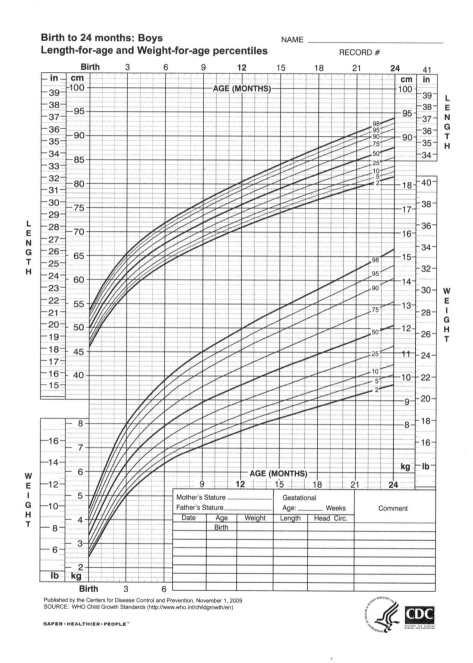

Birth to 24 months: Boys
Length-for-age and Weight-for-age percentiles

NAME _____

RECORD # _____

Published by the Centers for Disease Control and Prevention, November 1, 2009
SOURCE: WHO Child Growth Standards (http://www.who.int/childgrowth/en)

SAFER·HEALTHIER·PEOPLE™

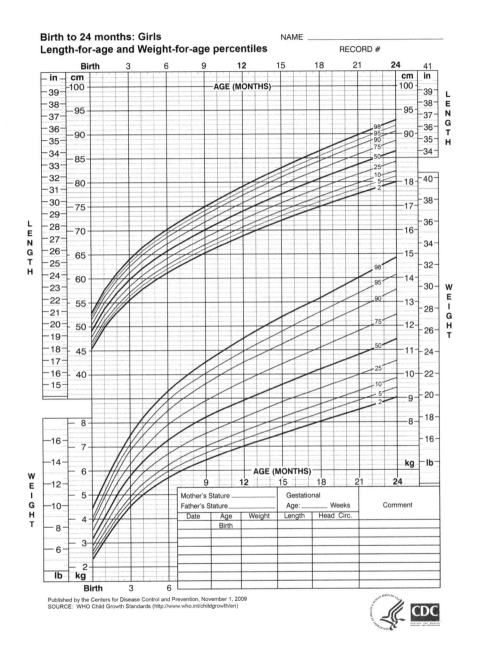

Birth to 24 months: Girls
Length-for-age and Weight-for-age percentiles

NAME _____

RECORD # _____

Published by the Centers for Disease Control and Prevention, November 1, 2009
SOURCE: WHO Child Growth Standards (http://www.who.int/childgrowth/en)

Tips for Avoiding Your Allergen

- All FDA-regulated manufactured food products that contain a "major food allergen" (milk, wheat, egg, peanuts, tree nuts, fish, crustacean shellfish, and soy) as an ingredient are required by U.S. law to list that allergen on the product label. For tree nuts, fish and crustacean shellfish, the specific type of nut or fish must be listed.
- Read all product labels carefully before purchasing and consuming any item.
- Be aware of unexpected sources of allergens, such as the ingredients listed below.
- *Note: This list does not imply that the allergen is always present in these foods; it is intended to serve as a reminder to always read the label and ask questions about ingredients.

 For a Milk-Free Diet

Avoid foods that contain milk or any of these ingredients:

butter, butter fat, butter oil, butter acid, butter ester(s)	lactalbumin, lactalbumin phosphate	solids, whole) milk protein hydrolysate pudding
buttermilk	lactoferrin	Recaldent®
casein	lactose	rennet casein
casein hydrolysate	lactulose	sour cream, sour cream
caseinates *(in all forms)*	milk *(in all forms,*	solids
cheese	*including condensed,*	sour milk solids
cottage cheese	*derivative, dry,*	tagatose
cream	*evaporated, goat's*	whey *(in all forms)*
curds	*milk and milk from*	whey protein
custard	*other animals, lowfat,*	hydrolysate
diacetyl	*malted, milkfat,*	yogurt
ghee	*nonfat, powder,*	
half-and-half	*protein, skimmed,*	

Milk is sometimes found in the following:

artificial butter flavor	culture and other	nisin
baked goods	bacterial cultures	nondairy products
caramel candies	luncheon meat, hot	nougat
chocolate	dogs, sausages	
lactic acid starter	margarine	

Keep the following in mind:

- Individuals who are allergic to cow's milk are often advised to also avoid milk from other domestic animals. For example, goat's milk protein is similar to cow's milk protein and may, therefore, cause a reaction in individuals who have a milk allergy.

 For a Wheat-Free Diet

Avoid foods that contain wheat or any of these ingredients:

bread crumbs	protein, instant,	semolina
bulgur	pastry, self-rising, soft	spelt
cereal extract	wheat, steel ground,	sprouted wheat
club wheat	stone ground, whole	triticale
couscous	wheat)	vital wheat gluten
cracker meal	hydrolyzed wheat	wheat (bran, durum,
durum	protein	germ, gluten, grass,
einkorn	Kamut®	malt, sprouts, starch)
emmer	matzoh, matzoh meal	wheat bran hydrolysate
farina	(also spelled as	wheat germ oil
flour (all purpose,	matzo, matzah, or	wheat grass
bread, cake, durum,	matza)	wheat protein isolate
enriched, graham,	pasta	whole wheat berries
high gluten, high	seitan	

Wheat is sometimes found in the following:

glucose syrup	soy sauce	surimi
oats	starch (gelatinized	
	starch, modified	
	starch, modified food	
	starch, vegetable	
	starch)	

 For an Egg-Free Diet

Avoid foods that contain eggs or any of these ingredients:

albumin (also spelled	livetin	vitellin
albumen)	lysozyme	words starting with
egg (dried, powdered,	mayonnaise	"ovo" or "ova" (such
solids, white, yolk)	meringue (meringue	as ovalbumin)
eggnog	powder)	
globulin	surimi	

Egg is sometimes found in the following:

baked goods	fried rice	meatloaf or meatballs
breaded items	ice cream	nougat
drink foam (alcoholic,	lecithin	pasta
specialty coffee)	marzipan	
egg substitutes	marshmallows	

Keep the following in mind:

- Individuals with egg allergy should also avoid eggs from duck, turkey, goose, quail, etc., as these are known to be cross-reactive with chicken egg.
- While the whites of an egg contain the allergenic proteins, patients with an egg allergy must avoid all eggs completely.

 For a Soy-Free Diet

Avoid foods that contain soy or any of these ingredients:

edamame	soy protein (concentrate, hydrolyzed,
miso	isolate)
natto	shoyu
soy (soy albumin, soy cheese, soy	soy sauce
fiber, soy flour, soy grits, soy ice	tamari
cream, soy milk, soy nuts, soy	tempeh
sprouts, soy yogurt)	textured vegetable protein (TVP)
soya	tofu
soybean (curd, granules)	

Soy is sometimes found in the following:

Asian cuisine	vegetable gum
vegetable broth	vegetable starch

Keep the following in mind:

- The FDA exempts highly refined soybean oil from being labeled as an allergen. Studies show most allergic individuals can safely eat soy oil that has been highly refined (not cold pressed, expeller pressed, or extruded soybean oil).
- Most individuals allergic to soy can safely eat soy lecithin.
- Follow your doctor's advice regarding these ingredients.

www.foodallergy.org

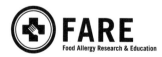

For a Shellfish-Free Diet

Avoid foods that contain shellfish or any of these ingredients:

barnacle	lobster (langouste,	prawns
crab	langoustine, Moreton	shrimp (crevette,
crawfish (crawdad,	bay bugs, scampi,	scampi)
crayfish, ecrevisse)	tomalley)	
krill		

! Mollusks are not considered major allergens under food labeling laws and may not be fully disclosed on a product label.

Your doctor may advise you to avoid mollusks or these ingredients:

abalone	limpet (lapas, opihi)	sea cucumber
clams (cherrystone,	mussels	sea urchin
geoduck, littleneck,	octopus	snails (escargot)
pismo, quahog)	oysters	squid (calamari)
cockle	periwinkle	whelk (Turban shell)
cuttlefish	scallops	

Shellfish are sometimes found in the following:

bouillabaisse	fish stock	surimi
cuttlefish ink	seafood flavoring (e.g.,	
glucosamine	crab or clam extract)	

Keep the following in mind:

- Any food served in a seafood restaurant may contain shellfish protein due to cross-contact.
- For some individuals, a reaction may occur from inhaling cooking vapors or from handling fish or shellfish.

For a Peanut-Free Diet

Avoid foods that contain peanuts or any of these ingredients:

artificial nuts	goobers	nut meat
beer nuts	ground nuts	peanut butter
cold pressed, expeller	mixed nuts	peanut flour
pressed, or extruded	monkey nuts	peanut protein
peanut oil	nut pieces	hydrolysate

Peanut is sometimes found in the following:

African, Asian	baked goods (e.g.,	enchilada sauce
(especially	pastries, cookies)	marzipan
Chinese, Indian,	candy (including	mole sauce
Indonesian, Thai,	chocolate candy)	nougat
and Vietnamese), and	chili	
Mexican dishes	egg rolls	

Keep the following in mind:

- Mandelonas are peanuts soaked in almond flavoring.
- The FDA exempts highly refined peanut oil from being labeled as an allergen. Studies show that most allergic individuals can safely eat peanut oil that has been highly refined (not cold pressed, expeller pressed, or extruded peanut oil). Follow your doctor's advice.
- A study showed that unlike other legumes, there is a strong possibility of cross-reaction between peanuts and lupine.
- Arachis oil is peanut oil.
- Many experts advise patients allergic to peanuts to avoid tree nuts as well.
- Sunflower seeds are often produced on equipment shared with peanuts.
- Some alternative nut butters, such as soy nut butter or sunflower seed butter, are produced on equipment shared with other tree nuts and, in some cases, peanuts. Contact the manufacturer before eating these products.

For a Tree-Nut-Free Diet

Avoid foods that contain nuts or any of these ingredients:

almond	hickory nut	nut pieces
artificial nuts	litchi/lichee/lychee nut	pecan
beechnut	macadamia nut	pesto
Brazil nut	marzipan/almond paste	pili nut
butternut	Nangai nut	pine nut (also referred
cashew	natural nut extract	to as Indian, pignoli,
chestnut	(e.g., almond, walnut)	pigñolia, pignon,
chinquapin nut	nut butters (e.g.,	piñon, and pinyon
coconut*	cashew butter)	nut)
filbert/hazelnut	nut meal	pistachio
gianduja (a chocolate-	nut meat	praline
nut mixture)	nut paste (e.g., almond	shea nut
ginkgo nut	paste)	walnut

Tree nuts are sometimes found in the following:

black walnut hull	nut distillates/alcoholic	walnut hull extract
extract (flavoring)	extracts	(flavoring)
natural nut extract	nut oils (e.g., walnut	
	oil, almond oil)	

Keep the following in mind:

- Mortadella may contain pistachios.
- There is no evidence that coconut oil and shea nut oil/butter are allergenic.
- Many experts advise patients allergic to tree nuts to avoid peanuts as well.
- Talk to your doctor if you find other nuts not listed here.
- Coconut, the seed of a drupaceous fruit, has typically not been restricted in the diets of people with tree nut allergy. However, in October of 2006, the FDA began identifying coconut as a tree nut. Medical literature documents a small number of allergic reactions to coconut; most occurred in people who were not allergic to other tree nuts. Ask your doctor if you need to avoid coconut.

For a Fish-Free Diet

Fish is sometimes found in the following:

barbecue sauce	fish oil	pizza (anchovy topping)
bouillabaisse	fish sauce imitation fish	roe
Caesar salad	or shellfish isinglass	salad dressing
caviar	lutefisk maw, maws	seafood flavoring
deep fried items	(fish maw)	shark cartilage
fish flavoring	fish stock	shark fin
fish flour	fishmeal	surimi
fish fume	nuoc mam (Vietnamese	sushi, sashimi
fish gelatin (kosher	name for fish sauce;	Worcestershire sauce
gelatin, marine	beware of other ethnic	
gelatin)	names)	

Keep the following in mind:

- If you have fish allergy, avoid seafood restaurants. Even if you order a non-fish item off of the menu, cross-contact of fish protein is possible.
- Asian cookery often uses fish sauce as a flavoring base. Exercise caution when eating this type of cuisine.
- Fish protein can become airborne in the steam released during cooking and may cause an allergic reaction. Stay away from cooking areas when fish is being prepared.

www.foodallergy.org
©2014, Food Allergy Research & Education (FARE)

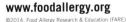

FARE
Food Allergy Research & Education

Helpful Websites for Parents

American Academy of Pediatrics (AAP)

www.healthychildren.org

www.aap.org

American Partnership for Eosinophilic Disorders

www.apfed.org

Celiac Disease Foundation

www.celiac.org

The Centers for Disease Control and Prevention (CDC)

www.cdc.gov

Ellyn Satter Institute

www.ellynsatterinstitute.org

Environmental Working Group

www.ewg.org

Food Allergy Research and Education

www.foodallergy.org/home

Gluten Free Drugs

www.glutenfreedrugs.com

Human Milk Banking Association of North America

www.hmbana.org

International Food Protein–Induced Enterocolitis Syndrome (FPIES) Association

www.fpies.org

North American Society of Pediatric Gastroenterology, Hepatology and Nutrition

www.gikids.org

United States Department of Agriculture (USDA)

www.choosemyplate.gov/

United States Department of Labor

www.dol.gov/whd/nursingmothers/faqbtnm.htm

United States Food and Drug Administration (FDA)

www.fda.gov/

About the Authors and Contributors

Dina M. DiMaggio

Dina is a board certified pediatrician at Pediatric Associates of NYC (where she met Liza and Susan), one of the oldest pediatric practices in Manhattan, and a clinical instructor at NYU Langone Medical Center. She has received numerous research awards, along with Patient's Choice Award (2008 to 2012) and compassionate doctor recognition (2010, 2012). She was featured in the *New York Times Magazine* as a Super Doctor in 2014 and in 2015 as a New York Rising Star. She is dedicated to educating parents on baby and toddler nutrition and gives talks to parent groups throughout New York.

She attended Barnard College (where she met Amanda), graduated summa cum laude and as a member of Phi Beta Kappa Society, and went on to attend medical school at Albert Einstein College of Medicine (with Amanda), where she was elected into the Alpha Omega Alpha Honor Society. She completed her pediatric residency at the Children's Hospital at Montefiore (where she met Anthony and Persephone) and her hematology/oncology fellowship at Memorial Sloan Kettering Cancer Center.

Anthony F. Porto

Anthony is a board-certified pediatrician and board certified pediatric gastroenterologist. He is an assistant professor of pediatrics and associate clinical chief of pediatric gastroenterology at Yale University and director, pediatric gastroenterology, at Greenwich Hospital in Greenwich, Connecticut. He is also the medical director of the Yale Pediatric Celiac Program. He sees patients in Greenwich, Trumbull, and New Haven, Connecticut. He has won numerous awards, including the Norman J. Seigel Award at Yale University in 2015 for leadership and providing outstanding clinical care, as well as Physician of the Year during his time at Morgan Stanley Children's Hospital. He has been named Castle Connolly Top Doctors since 2012. He is on the American Academy of Pediatrics PREP Gastroenterology Advisory Board and a member of the North American Society of Pediatric Gastroenterology and Hepatology's Public Education Committee and writes web-based educational materials. Anthony is interested in nutrition, especially in the care of children with difficulty gaining weight, feeding issues, and celiac disease. He loves teaching and educating parents and gives lectures to parents throughout Connecticut.

He graduated from Columbia University with a bachelor of arts in neuroscience and behavior and attended medical school at Tufts University School of Medicine, where he also received his master of public health. He completed his pediatric residency at the Children's Hospital at Montefiore Medical Center (where he met Dina and Persephone) and his pediatric gastroenterology fellowship at the Morgan Stanley Children's Hospital of New York at Columbia University (where he met Janet).

Amanda Cox

Amanda Cox is board certified in pediatrics and in allergy and immunology. From 2008 to 2014, she was an assistant professor of pediatrics on the medical faculty of the Icahn School of Medicine at Mount Sinai, where she worked at the Jaffe Food Allergy Institute, which is renowned for patient care and groundbreaking research in the field of pediatric food allergy. She has gained special expertise in caring for infants, children, and adolescents who have severe and extensive food allergic issues. She also currently is the president of the New York Allergy and Asthma Society and is an involved member of the American Academy of Allergy, Asthma & Immunology, where she also serves on the Adverse Reactions to Foods Committee. In 2014, Amanda joined ProHEALTH Care Associates to practice pediatric allergy and immunology in Brooklyn, New York.

Amanda graduated cum laude from Columbia University (where she met Anthony and Dina) with a bachelor of arts in American history, and attended Albert Einstein College of Medicine (with Dina). She completed her residency in pediatrics as well as a fellowship in allergy and immunology at the North Shore Long Island Jewish Medical Center.

Persephone Jones

Persephone is a board-certified developmental-behavioral pediatrician. She is the chief of the Division of Developmental Medicine at Nemours /Alfred I. duPont Hospital for Children in Wilmington, Delaware. She sees patients in Wilmington, Delaware, and Voorhees, New Jersey. Persephone graduated from Rutgers University with a bachelor of arts in biology and psychology, and completed medical school at Rutgers New Jersey Medical School. She completed her pediatric residency at the Children's Hospital at Montefiore, where she met Dina and Anthony. Persephone completed her fellowship in developmental-behavioral pediatrics at Boston Children's Hospital during which time she earned a master of public health from the Harvard School of Public Health.

Janet Kopchinski

Janet is a pediatric dietitian and board-certified nutrition support dietitian. She is a private practice dietitian at Be Well, a Wellness Center in Morristown, New Jersey. She previously worked for over ten years at the Morgan Stanley Children's Hospital of New York-Presbyterian (where she met Anthony). Janet worked there as the lead dietitian of the adolescent bariatric surgery and medical obesity program. She also gained a vast amount of experience working with children with poor weight gain, too much weight gain, food allergies, and other nutritional issues.

Susan Berger

Susan is a board-certified lactation consultant and has a doctorate in international nutrition. She fell in love with international work in 1980 when she served as a Peace Corps Volunteer in the Democratic Republic of Congo. She worked in dozens of countries in Africa, South-East Asia, and South America as Director of Nutrition for Helen Keller International and as a consultant to organizations such as the United Nations Children's Fund, the World Bank, the World Health Organization, the Centers for Disease Control and Prevention, and the International Red Cross. She has worked in a private lactation practice since 2002 and served for seven years as a board member of the New York Lactation Consultant Association.

Alison Gütwaks

Alison is a personal chef, recipe developer, and blogger. Alison started her company, AliBabka, in 2013 with a focus on providing personalized menus. She specializes in coming up with creative options for those with dietary restrictions, such as food allergies and kosher restrictions. She believes that anyone can cook with a little direction, the correct tools, and the right amount of patience.

Chef Alison graduated with a degree in culinary arts from the prestigious Institute of Culinary Education (ICE) in Manhattan. She has been featured in the Wall Street Journal. She has over fifteen years of experience working as a chocolatier and sous chef. Alison is a former chef and event planner for Celebrations Kosher Catering in East Hanover, New Jersey, where she helped spearhead the catering company's opening with her innovative and fresh ideas and was the corporate recipe developer for OSEM USA, an Israeli-based food company.

Dini Klein

Dini is an enthusiastic foodie, personal chef, working mother, and the founder of Dini Delivers. The demand for homemade authentic and delicious food led to the start of a completely customized food delivery service. As a working mom, Dini understands the struggle mothers face when it comes to feeding their children healthy and delicious food. Dini makes it simple.

Dini graduated from the Fashion Institute of Technology and realized she craved food more than fashion. She graduated from the Center of Kosher Culinary Arts (CKCA) in 2011 with a Servsafe certification, and followed up her training with an externship at The Prime Grill.

Medical Reviewer: Liza Natale

Liza is a general pediatrician with Pediatric Associates of NYC in midtown Manhattan. She has been in practice there since 2004. Liza is a graduate of Kenyon College and SUNY Health Science Center at Brooklyn. She completed her pediatric residency and chief residency at NYU Medical Center/Bellevue Hospital. In addition, Liza serves as a pediatric consultant to the 92 Street Y's Parenting Center and facilitates workshops there on such topics as sleep, starting solids, and baby care for expectant parents.

Acknowledgments

We would like to thank everyone who made this book possible.

Our mentors at the Children Hospital at Montefiore, Memorial Sloan Kettering Cancer Center, Columbia University, Yale University, and Pediatric Associates of NYC, we thank you for teaching us how to practice the art and science of medicine and that being a pediatrician was never a nine-to-five job but a dedicated lifestyle.

Sharon, our agent, for responding to our frequent emails, answering our many questions, and guiding us through the publishing process. We can't thank you enough for believing in us and being our enthusiastic supporter.

Kelly, our editor, for keeping us on track, always being available, and for her guidance and dedication each step of the way. For our hardworking team at Ten Speed for organizing our thoughts into a real book.

Amy Ciner, for being our constant sounding board and best friend throughout this process, reviewing our recipes and putting us in contact with our chefs.

Jane Lee, for reviewing the recipe portions of our book, her friendship, offering her advice and for supporting us through the publishing process from the beginning when this book was only an idea. We love your lasagna and cookie recipes!

Dina:

Anthony, we instantly clicked as soon as we met in residency and we will always be "two peds in a pod" no matter what ups and downs face us. I'm grateful to have you as my partner and best friend and together to having never given up on our vision becoming a reality. High-Hoo!

To my father who is my hero and has worked twelve hours or more a day for fifty years as a butcher so that he could provide my sisters and me with an education. He has taught us the values of hard work, honesty, and a thirst for knowledge. To my mother, who has always been the definition of unconditional love and kindness and a constant support for whenever my family and I needed her. To my sisters, for their constant support and for allowing me to use my adorable niece and nephew as guinea pigs throughout this process. And to my nanny, Ancilla Jones, my in-laws (Marsha, Val, Casey, and the rest of the Walters), and my friends and colleagues of PANYC (Christina, Michael, Beth, Emily, Liz, Nina, Jaz, Pam, Gabby, and Brianna) for eating and then eating over and over again the recipes until we got them just right.

To Derek, my husband, for being my voice of reason, for giving me my happily-ever-after, and for each day teaching me how to be a better parent through his actions.

My daughters, Julia and Evelyn, you are my everythings. Thank you for making me a better person. You showed me I didn't know what love was until I held you. I only hope I can be as good of a mother to you as my mother is to me.

Anthony:

Dina, I can't believe that this idea that popped up while we were on the phone one day actually ended up as a book. What a journey it has been! Hey ooh!! I could not have imagined experiencing it with anyone else and feel fortunate to have you as my partner and best friend.

My dad for always being there for me—driving me to school, moving me in and out of my college dorm, coming with me to my medical school interviews, and always "waiting for Anthony" whenever I was late (which was often). Thanks for driving the tester recipes to Connecticut for me to taste. You are an amazing father and grandfather.

To my sister, Irene, who has been my biggest fan since I can remember. Thanks for all of your words of encouragement, constant enthusiasm, and continued support.

A special thanks to my mother who always taught me to enjoy the little things in life. I think about and miss you every day. You are Sebby's guardian angel.

To Lisa, my mother-in-law, for testing the recipes in this book and offering her suggestions. To John, my father-in-law, for helping us organize our LLC and for his enthusiastic lectures on everyday economics. Sebby is lucky to have such a great Grandma and Pop! To Lizzie and Laura, thanks for taking such good care of Sebby and for sending me pictures of him while I am at work.

My husband, John, who grounds me in life. Thanks for your love and support always, for reading through early and late drafts, always understanding when I was cranky and when I had a last minute deadline or a phone call with Dina. I could not have written this book without you. Thanks for being the best papa to our son.

My son, Sebby, for changing my life in the best way possible. You sat on my lap while I was typing and editing parts of the book. Thanks for making me smile every day and making me understand what is truly important.

References

Chapter One: 0 to 3 Months

1. American Academy of Pediatrics. "Developmental Milestones: 1 Month." HealthyChildren.org. http://www.healthychildren.org/English/ages-stages/baby/Pages/Developmental-Milestones-1-Month.aspx (accessed June 9, 2015).

2. The Academy of Breastfeeding Medicine. "ABM Clinical Protocol # 8: Human Milk Storage Information for Home Use for Full-term Infants Breastfeeding Medicine." Breastfeeding Medicine no. 3 (March 2010): 127–130.

3. The Academy of Breastfeeding Medicine. "ABM Clinical Protocol #34: Allergic Proctocolitis in the Exclusively Breastfed Infant." Breastfeeding Medicine no. 6 (December 2011): 435–40.

4. American Academy of Pediatrics. "Pacifiers: Satisfying Your Baby's Needs." HealthyChildren.org. http://www.healthychildren.org/English/ages-stages/baby/crying-colic/Pages/Pacifiers-Satisfying-Your-Babys-Needs.aspx (accessed June 9, 2015).

5. American Academy of Pediatrics. "Breastfeeding and the Use of Human Milk." *Pediatrics* no. 3 (March 2012): e827–841.

6. American Academy of Pediatrics. "Introducing the Bottle." HealthyChildren.org. http://www.healthychildren.org/English/ages-stages/baby/breastfeeding/Pages/Introducing-the-Bottle.aspx (accessed June 9, 2015).

7. American Academy of Allergy Asthma & Immunology. "Anaphylaxis." aaaai.org. http://www.aaaai.org/conditions-and-treatments/conditions-a-to-z-search/Anaphylaxis.aspx (accessed June 9, 2015).

8. American Academy of Pediatrics. "How to Safely Prepare Formula with Water." HealthyChildren.org. https://www.healthychildren.org/English/ages-stages/baby/feeding-nutrition/Pages/How-to-Safely-Prepare-Formula-with-Water.aspx (accessed June 9, 2015).

9. American Academy of Pediatrics. "Transitional Milk and Mature Milk." healthychildren.org. http://www.healthychildren.org/English/ages-stages/baby/breastfeeding/Pages/Transitional-Milk-and-Mature-Milk.aspx (accessed June 9, 2015).

10. American Academy of Pediatrics. "Is Your Drinking Water Safe?" healthychildren.org. http://www.healthychildren.org/English/safety-prevention/all-around/Pages/Is-Your-Drinking-Water-Safe.aspx (accessed June 9, 2015).

11. American Academy of Pediatrics and the Section on Breastfeeding and Committee on Nutrition. "Prevention of Rickets and Vitamin D Deficiency in Infants, Children, and Adolescents" *Pediatrics*, no 4. (November 2008) 1142–52.

12. American Academy of Pediatrics. "Vitamin & Iron Supplements." healthychildren.org. http://www.healthychildren.org/English/ages-stages/baby/feeding-nutrition/Pages/Vitamin-Iron-Supplements.aspx.

13. American Academy of Pediatrics. "FAQ: Fluoride and Children." healthychildren.org. http://www.healthychildren.org/English/healthy-living/oral-health/Pages/FAQ-Fluoride-and-Children.aspx (accessed June 9, 2015).

14. American Dental Association. "Fluoride and Infant Formula FAQ." ada.org. http://www.ada.org/en/public-programs/advocating-for-the-public/fluoride-and-fluoridation/ recent-fluoridation-issues/infant-formula-and-fluoridated-water/fluoride-and-infant-formula-faq (accessed June 9, 2015).

15. Atanaskovic-Markovic, M. "Refractory Proctocolitis in the Exclusively Breastfed Infants." *Endocrine, Metabolic & Immune Disorders—Drug Targets,* no. 14. 63–66.

16. Berg, J, and Gerweck, C. "Evidence-Based Clinical Recommendations Regarding Fluoride Intake from Reconstituted Infant Formula and Enamel Fluorosis: A Report of the American Dental Association Council on Scientific Affairs." *The Journal of the American Dental Association* no. 1 (January 2011): 79–87.

17. Boyce, et al. "Guidelines for the Diagnosis and Management of Food Allergy in the United States: Summary of the NIAID-Sponsored Expert Panel Report." *JACI* no. 6 (December 2010): 1105–18.

18. Centers for Disease Control and Prevention. "Proper Handling and Storage of Human Milk." cdc.gov. http://www.cdc.gov/breastfeeding/recommendations/ handling_breastmilk.htm (accessed June 9, 2015).

19. Centers for Disease Control and Prevention. "Vitamin D Supplementation." cdc.gov. http://www.cdc.gov/breastfeeding/recommendations/vitamin_d.htm (accessed June 9, 2015).

20. Centers for Disease Control and Prevention. "Overview: Infant Formula and Fluorosis. cdc.gov. http://www.cdc.gov/fluoridation/safety/infant_formula.htm (accessed June 9, 2015).

21. Centers for Disease Control and Prevention. "Calcium and Bone Health." cdc.gov. http://www.cdc.gov/nutrition/everyone/basics/vitamins/calcium.html (accessed June 9, 2015).

22. Consumer Reports. "Baby formula buying guide." consumerreports.org. http://www.consumerreports.org/cro/baby-formula/buying-guide.htm (accessed June 9, 2015).

23. Consumer Reports. "Baby Bottle Buying Guide." consumerreports.org. http:// www.consumerreports.org/cro/baby-bottles/buying-guide.htm (accessed June 9, 2015).

24. Dr. Brown's. "Dr. Brown's Nipples." drbrownsbaby.com. http://www.drbrownsbaby .com/bottles-accessories/nipples (accessed June 9, 2015).

25. Enfamil. "Help Advice and Answers: Why are storage instructions different for your liquid and powder formulas?" Enfamil.com. http://www.enfamil.com/ help-advice-answers/faq?&page=7 (accessed June 9, 2015).

26. Fleischer et al. "Primary Prevention of Allergic Disease Through Nutritional Interventions." *JACI* no. 1 (January 2013): 29–36.

27. Johns Hopkins Hospital, Jason Robertson, Nicole Shilkofski. *The Harriet Lane Handbook,* 17th edition. Philadelphia, PA: Elsevier Mosby, 2005.

28. Keim, SA, et al. "Microbial Contamination of Human Milk Purchased Via the Internet." *Pediatrics* no. 5 (November 2013): e1227-e1235.

29. Keim, SA, et al. "Cow's Milk Contamination of Human Milk Purchased via the Internet." *Pediatrics* no. 5 (May 2015).

30. Kleinman, RE, et al. and the AAP Committee on Nutrition. "The use of whole cow's milk in infancy." *Pediatrics* no. 6, part 1 (June 1992): 1105–9.

31. Koletzko, B, Poindexter, B, and Uauy, R. *World Review of Nutrition and Dietetics Nutritional Care of the Premature Infant.* Basel, Switzerland: Karger, 2014.

32. Kramer, MS, and Kakuma, R. "Optimal duration of exclusive breastfeeding." *Cochrane Database Syst Review* no. 8 (August 2012).

33. La Leche League International. "What are the LLLI guidelines for storing my pumped milk?" llli.org. http://www.llli.org/faq/milkstorage.html (accessed June 9, 2015).

34. La Leche League International. "How Do I Wean My Baby?" llli.org. http://www.lalecheleague.org/faq/weanhowto.html (accessed June 9, 2015).

35. La Leche League International. "Maternal Nutrition During Breastfeeding." llli.org. http://www.llli.org/nb/nbmarapr04p44.html (accessed June 9, 2015).

36. Mayo Clinic. "Diseases and Conditions: Premature Birth." mayoclinic.org. http://www.mayoclinic.org/diseases-conditions/premature-birth/basics/definition/CON-20020050 (accessed June 9, 2015).

37. Perrin, M, et al. "A mixed-methods observational study of human milk sharing communities on Facebook." *Breastfeed Med* no. 9 (April 2014): 128–134.

38. "Pregnant and Breastfeeding Mom Daily Meal Plan." www.choosemyplate.gov; (accessed June 9, 2015)

39. Sexton, S, and Natale, R. "Risks and Benefits of Pacifiers." *Am Fam Physician* no. 8 (April 2009): 681–685.

40. Shelov, S. *AAP Caring for your baby and young child, Birth to age 5* 4th Edition. New York: Random House, 2004.

41. Silverman, WA, ed. *Dunham's Premature Infants, 3rd edition.* New York: Hoeber, Inc., Medical Division of Harper and Brothers, 1961, pp. 143–144.

42. Texas Children's Hospital, Houston. *Texas Children's Hospital Pediatric Nutrition Reference Guide 10th edition.* Houston, Texas: Texas Children's Hospital, February 2014.

43. United States Department of Agriculture Food and Nutrition Service. "Infant Feeding Guide." wicworks.nal.usda.gov. http://wicworks.nal.usda.gov/infants/infant-feeding-guide (accessed June 9, 2015).

44. United States Department of Health & Human Services. "Use of Donor Human Milk." fda.org. http://www.fda.gov/ScienceResearch/SpecialTopics/PediatricTherapeutics Research/ucm235203.htm (accessed June 9, 2015).

45. United States Department of Agriculture. "Eating Fish While You Are Pregnant or Breastfeeding." choosemyplate.gov http://www.choosemyplate.gov/pregnancy-breastfeeding/eating-fish.html (accessed June 9, 2015).

46. United States Department of Agriculture. "Tips for Breastfeeding Moms." nal.usda.gov. http://www.nal.usda.gov/wicworks/Topics/BreastfeedingFactSheet.pdf (accessed June 9, 2015).

47. V Bouvard, D Loomis, et al. On behalf of the International Agency for Research on Cancer Monograph Working Group. "Carcinogenicity of consumption of red and processed meat." Published Online: 26 October 2015. The Lancet Oncology.

48. "A Comprehensive Overview of Store Brand Infant Formula" *Consultant for Pediatricians*, supplement (February 2014): 1–8.

Chapter Two: 4 to 6 Months

1. American Academy of Pediatrics. "AAP Offers Advice for Parents Concerned About Arsenic in Food." aap.org. http://www.aap.org/en-us/about-the-aap/aap-press-room/Pages/AAP-Offers-Advice-For-Parents-Concerned-About-Arsenic-in-Food.aspx (accessed June 9, 2015).

2. American Academy of Pediatric Dentistry. "Frequently Asked Questions." aapd.org. http://www.aapd.org/resources/frequently_asked_questions/#36 (accessed June 9, 2015).

3. American Academy of Pediatrics. "Vegetarian Diets for Children. healthychildren.org. http://www.healthychildren.org/English/age-stages/gradeschool/nutrition/Pages/ Vegetartian-Diet- for-Children.aspx (accessed June 9, 2015).

4. American Academy of Pediatrics. *Red Book: 2012 Report of the Committee on Infectious Diseases.* Pickering LK, ed. 29th ed. Elk Grove Village, IL: American Academy of Pediatrics, 2012.

5. American Academy of Pediatrics Committee on Environmental Health. "Infant methemoglobinemia: the role of dietary nitrate in food and water." *Pediatrics* no. 3 (September 2005): 784–6.

6. American Academy of Pediatrics. "Water & Juice." healthychildren.org. http://www.healthychildren.org/English/ages-stages/baby/feeding-nutrition/Pages/ Water-Juice.aspx. (accessed June 9, 2015).

7. American Heart Association. "Vegetarian Diets." heart.org. http://www.heart.org/ HEARTORG/GettingHealthy/NutritionCenter/Vegetarian-Diets_UCM_306032_Article .jsp# (accessed June 9, 2015).

8. Baker RD, Greer, FR. Committee on Nutrition, American Academy of Pediatrics. "Diagnosis and prevention of iron deficiency and iron-deficiency anemia in infants and young children (0–3 years of age)." *Pediatrics* (November 2010); 126(5): 1040-50.

9. Boyce, J, Assa'ad, A, Burks, AW, et al. "NIAID-Sponsored Expert Panel. Guidelines for the Diagnosis and Management of Food Allergy in the United States: Summary of the NIAID-Sponsored Expert Panel Report." *J Allergy Clin Immunol* no. 6 (December 2010): 1105–18.

10. Brady, MT, and Byington, CL. Committees on Infectious Disease and Nutrition, American Academy of Pediatrics. "Consumption of Raw or Unpasteurized Milk and Milk Products by Pregnant Women and Children." *Pediatrics* no. 1 (January 2014): 175–79.

11. Cameron, S , Heath, A, and Taylor, R. "How Feasible Is Baby-Led Weaning as an Approach to Infant Feeding? A Review of the Evidence." *Nutrients* no. 4 (November 2012): 1575–1609.

12. Centers for Disease Control and Prevention. "Iron and Iron Deficiency." cdc.gov. http://www.cdc.gov/nutrition/everyone/basics/vitamins/iron.html (accessed June 9, 2015).

13. Chan TY. "Vegetable-borne nitrate and nitrite and the risk of methaemoglobiaemia." *Toxicol Lett* no. 1–2 (January 2011): 107–8.

14. Children's Hospital Colorado. "Stools—Unusual Color." childrenscolorado.org. http://www.childrenscolorado.org/wellness-safety/pediatric/stoolscolor/ stools—unusual-color (accessed June 9, 2015).

15. Consumer Reports. "Arsenic in Your Food." consumerreports.org. http://consumerreports.org/cro/magazine/2012/11/arsenic-in-your-food/index.htm (accessed June 9, 2015).

16. Craig, WJ, and Mangels, AR. "Position of the American Dietetic Association: Vegetarian diets." *Journal of the American Dietetic Association* no. 7 (July 2009): 1266–1282.

17. Du Toit, G, Roberts, G, et al. "Randomized Trial of Peanut Consumption in Infants at Risk for Peanut Allergy." *NEJM* no. 9 (February 2015): 803–813.

18. Environmental Working Group. "EWG's 2015 Shopper's Guide to Pesticides in Produce." ewg.org. http://www.ewg.org/foodnews/ (accessed June 9, 2015).

19. Fleischer et al. "Primary Prevention of Allergic Disease Through Nutritional Interventions." *JACI* no. 1 (January 2013): 29–36.

20. Forman, J, Silverstein, J, Committee on Nutrition and Council on Environmental Health. "Clinical Report: Organic Foods: Health and Environmental Advantages and Disadvantages." *Pediatrics* no. 5 (November 2012): e1406–15.

21. Fregusson, DM, Horwood, LJ, Shannon, FT. "Early solid feeding and recurrent childhood eczema: A 10-year longitudinal study." *Pediatrics no.* 4 (October 1990): 541–6.

22. Greer, F, Sicherer, S, Burks, W, and the Committee on Nutrition and Section on Allergy and Immunology. "Effects of Early Nutritional Interventions on the Development of Atopic Disease in Infants and Children: The Role of Maternal Dietary Restriction, Breastfeeding, Timing of Introduction of Complementary Foods, and Hydrolyzed Formulas." *Pediatrics* no. 1 (January 2008), 183–191.

23. Greer, FR, Shannon, M, American Academy of Pediatrics Committee on Nutrition, Huh, S, and Rifas-Shiman S, et al. "Timing of Solid Food Introduction and Risk of Obesity in Pre-School Aged Children." *Pediatrics* no. 127(3) (March 2011): e544–51.

24. Johns Hopkins Hospital, Jason Robertson, Nicole Shilkofski. *The Harriet Lane Handbook*, 17th edition. Philadelphia, PA: Elsevier Mosby, 2005.

25. Macknin, ML, and Medendorp, SV, et al. "Infant sleep and bedtime cereal." *Am J Dis Child* no. 9 (September 1989): 1066–8.

26. Mayo Clinic. "Healthy Lifestyle: Infant and Toddler Health." mayoclinic.org. http://www.mayoclinic.org/healthy-lifestyle/infant-and-toddler-health/expert-answers/infant-growth/faq-20058037 (accessed June 9, 2015).

27. Pediatr Gastroenterol Nutr. "Complementary feeding: a commentary by the ESPGHAN Committee on Nutrition." Agostoni C1, Decsi T, Fewtrell M, Goulet O, Kolacek S, Koletzko B, Michaelsen KF, Moreno L, Puntis J, Rigo J, Shamir R, Szajewska H, Turck D, van Goudoever J; ESPGHAN Committee on Nutrition: 2008 Jan;46(1): 99–110.

28. Sampson, HA, and Bernstein, D, et al. "Food allergy: a practice parameter update." *J Allergy Clin Immunol* no. 5 (November 2014): 1016–25.

29. St. Vincent Healthcare. "The Paleo Diet." svh-mt.org. http://www.svh-mt.org/services-and-departments/pediatrics-st-vincent-childrens-healthcare/fortin-pediatric-specialty-clinic/pediatric-gastrointestinal-clinic/gi-spotlight/the-paleo-diet/ (accessed June 9, 2015).

30. Texas Children's Hospital, Houston. *Texas Children's Hospital Pediatric Nutrition Reference Guide 10th edition*. Houston, Texas: Texas Children's Hospital, February 2014.

31. United States Department of Agriculture. "Basics for Handling Food Safely." http://www.fsis.usda.gov/wps/portal/fsis/topics/food-safety-education/get-answers/food-safety-fact-sheets/safe-food-handling/basics-for-handling-food-safely/ct_index (accessed June 9, 2015).

32. United States Food and Drug Administration. "Questions & Answers: Apple Juice and Arsenic." fda.gov. http://www.fda.gov/Food/ResourcesForYou/Consumers/ucm271595.htm (accessed June 9, 2015).

33. United States Food and Drug Administration. "The Dangers of Raw Milk: Unpasteurized Milk Can Pose a Serious Health Risk." fda.gov. http://www.fda.gov/Food/ResourcesForYou/Consumers/ucm079516.htm (accessed June 9, 2015).

34. United States Food and Drug Administration. "Food Safety for Moms to Be: Once Baby Arrives." http://www.fda.gov/Food/ResourcesForYou/HealthEducators/ucm089629.htm (accessed June 9, 2015).

35. United States Department of Agriculture. "Infant Nutrition and Feeding Guide for Use in the WIC and CSF Programs." nal.usda.gov. http://wicworks.nal.usda.gov/infants/infant-feeding-guide (accessed June 9, 2015).

36. Vriezinga, SL, and Auricchop, R, et al. "Randomized feeding intervention in infants at high risk for celiac disease." *NEJM* no. 14 (October 2014): 1304–15.

Chapter Three: 7 to 8 months

1. American Academy of Pediatrics. "Developmental Milestones: 7 Months." healthychildren.org. http://www.healthychildren.org/English/agesstages/baby/Pages/Developmental-Milestones-7-Months.aspx (accessed June 9, 2015).

2. American Academy of Pediatrics. "Amber Teething Necklaces: A Caution for Parents." https://www.healthychildren.org/English/ages-stages/baby/teething-tooth-care/Pages/Amber-Teething-Necklaces.aspx (Accessed June 9, 2015).

3. American Academy of Pediatrics. "Diarrhea." https://www.healthychildren.org/English/health-issues/conditions/abdominal/Pages/Diarrhea.aspx (Accessed June 9, 2015).

4. Eunice Kennedy Shriver National Institute of Child Health and Human Development. "What are the DGAs for Moms & Infants?" nichd.nih.gov. http://www.nichd.nih.gov/health/topics/breastfeeding/conditioninfo/Pages/dga.aspx#calories (accessed June 9, 2015).

5. Food Allergy Research & Education. "Food Allergen Labeling and Consumer Protection Act." foodallergy.org. http://www.foodallergy.org/laws-and-regulations/falcpa (accessed June 9, 2015).

6. Lionetti, E, and Casetellaneta, et al. "Introduction of Gluten, HLA Status, and the Risk of Celiac Disease of Children." *NEJM* no. 371 (October 2014): 1295–1303.

7. Maharshak, N, and Shapiro, J, et al. "Carotenoderma—a review of the current literature." *International Journal of Dermatology* no. 3 (March 2003): 178–181.

8. Mayo Clinic. "Infant Development: Milestones from 7 to 9 Months." mayoclinic.org, http://www.mayoclinic.org/healthy-living/infant-and-toddler-health/in-depth/infant-development/art-20047086 (accessed June 9, 2015).

9. Mohrbacher, N, and Stock, J. *The Breastfeeding Answer Book*, Chicago, IL: La Leche League International, 2012.

10. Texas Children's Hospital, Houston. *Texas Children's Hospital Pediatric Nutrition Reference Guide 10th edition*. Houston, Texas: Texas Children's Hospital, February 2014.

11. United States Department of Agriculture. "Basics for Handling Food Safely." fsis.usda.gov. http://www.fsis.usda.gov/wps/portal/fsis/topics/food-safety-education/get-answers/food-safety-fact-sheets/safe-food-handling/basics-for-handling-food-safely/ct_index (accessed June 9, 2015).

12. United States Food and Drug Administration. "Hyland Teething Tablets: Questions and Answers." fda.gov. http://www.fda.gov/forconsumers/consumerupdates/ucm230762.htm (accessed June 9, 2015).

13. United States Food and Drug Administration. "Benzocaine and Babies: Not a Good Mix." fda.gov. http://www.fda.gov/forconsumers/consumerupdates/ucm306062.htm (accessed June 9, 2015).

14. United States Food and Drug Administration. "Hyland's Teething Tablets: Recall—Risk of Harm to Children." fda.gov. http://www.fda.gov/Safety/MedWatch/SafetyInformation/SafetyAlertsforHumanMedicalProducts/ucm230764.htm (accessed June 9, 2015).

15. United States Food and Drug Administration. "Benzocaine Topical Products: Sprays, Gels, and Liquids—Risk of Methemoglobinemia." fda.gov. http://www.fda.gov/safety/medwatch/safetyinformation/safetyalertsforhumanmedicalproducts/ucm250264.htm (accessed June 9, 2015).

16. Volta, U, and Bardell, MT, et al. "An Italian prospective multicenter survey on patients suspected of having non-celiac gluten sensitivity." *BMC Medicine* no. 12 (May 2014).

17. Vriezinga, SL, and Auricchop, R, et al. "Randomized feeding intervention in infants at high risk for celiac disease." *NEJM* no. 14 (October 2014): 1304–15.

Chapter Four: 9 to 12 Months

1. American Academy of Pediatrics. "Responding to a Choking Emergency." healthychildren.org. http://www.healthychildren.org/English/health-issues/injuries-emergencies/Pages/Responding-to-a-Choking-Emergency.aspx (accessed June 9, 2015).

2. American Academy of Pediatrics (AAP) radio series "A Minute for Kids," http://www.aap.org/en-us/about-the-aap/aap-press-room/aap-press-room-media-center/Pages/Anemia.aspx#sthash.RUuycEzz.dpuf (accessed June 9, 2015).

3. Chapin, MM, and Rochette, LM. "Nonfatal choking on food among children 14 years or younger in the United States, 2001–2009." *Pediatrics* no. 2 (August 2013): 275–81.

4. Centers for Disease Control and Prevention. "Dietary Sources of Iron." cdc.gov. http://www.cdc.gov/nutrition/everyone/basics/vitamins/iron.html#Iron%20Sources (accessed June 9, 2015).

5. Centers for Disease Control and Prevention. "Iron and Iron Deficiency." cdc.gov. http://www.cdc.gov/nutrition/everyone/basics/vitamins/iron.html (accessed June 9, 2015).

6. Committee on Injury, Violence, and Poison Prevention. "Prevention of Choking Among Children." *Pediatrics* no. 3 (March 2010): 601–7.

7. Duro, D, and Duggan, C. "The BRAT Diet for Acute Diarrhea in Children: Should It Be Used?" *Practical Gastroenterology* no. 51 (June 2007): 60, 65–68.

8. Grohskopf, LA, and Olsen, SJ. "Prevention and Control of Seasonal Influenza with Vaccines: Recommendations of the Advisory Committee on Immunization Practices (ACIP)—United States, 2014–15 Influenza Season" *MMWR* no. 32. (August 2014): 691-697.

9. Johns Hopkins Hospital, Brandon Engorn, and Jamie Fierlage. *The Harriet Lane Handbook,* 20th Edition. Philadelphia, PA: Elsevier Mosby, 2014.

10. King, CK, and Glass, R, et al. "Managing acute gastroenteritis among children: oral rehydration, maintenance, and nutritional therapy." *MMWR Recomm Rep.* no 52. (November 2003): 1–16.

11. Kleinman, R. *Pediatric Nutrition Handbook, 6th edition.* Elk Grove Village, IL: American Academy of Pediatrics, 2009.

12. Muensterer, O. "Infant Botulism." *Pediatrics in Review* no. 12 (December 2000): 427.

13. Texas Children's Hospital, Houston. *Texas Children's Hospital Pediatric Nutrition Reference Guide 10th edition.* Houston, Texas: Texas Children's Hospital, February 2014

14. United States Department of Agriculture. "DRI Tablets and Application Reports." http://fnic.nal.usda.gov/dietary-guidance/dietary-reference-intakes/dri-tables-and-application-reports (accessed June 9, 2015).

Chapter Five: The Toddler Years

1. American Academy of Pediatrics Section on Breastfeeding Policy Statement. "Breastfeeding and the Use of Human Milk." *Pediatrics* no. 3 (February 2012): e827–e841.

2. American Academy of Pediatrics. "Avoiding Trans Fats." healthychildren.org. https://www.healthychildren.org/English/healthy-living/nutrition/Pages/Avoiding-Trans-Fats.aspx (accessed June 9, 2015).

3. American Academy of Pediatrics. "What About Fat and Cholesterol?" healthychildren.org. http://www.healthychildren.org/English/healthy-living/nutrition/Pages/What-About-Fat-And-Cholesterol.aspx (accessed June 9, 2015).

4. American Academy of Pediatrics. "Self-Feeding." healthychildren.org. http://www.healthychildren.org/English/ages-stages/toddler/nutrition/Pages/Self-Feeding.aspx (accessed June 9, 2015).

5. American Cancer Society. "The Bottom Line on Soy and Breast Cancer Risk." cancer.org. http://www.cancer.org/cancer/news/expertvoices/post/2012/08/02/the-bottom-line-on-soy-and-breast-cancer-risk.aspx (accessed June 9, 2015).

6. American Heart Association. "Dietary Recommendations for Healthy Children." heart.org. http://www.heart.org/HEARTORG/GettingHealthy/Dietary-Recommendations-for-Healthy-Children_UCM_303886_Article.jsp (accessed June 9, 2015).

7. Baker, SS, and Baker, RD. "Early Exposure to Dietary Sugar and Salt." *Pediatrics* no. 3. (March 2015): 550–551.

8. Behrman, Richard, Robert Kliegman, and Hal Jenson. *Nelson Textbook of Pediatrics, 16th edition.* Philadelphia, PA: W. B. Saunders Company, 2000.

9. Bhatia, J, Greer, F, and the American Academy of Pediatrics Committee on Nutrition. "Use of Soy Protein–Based Formulas in Infant Feeding." *Pediatrics* no. 5 (May 2008): 1062-68.

10. Blue Diamond Almond Breeze. "Almond Milk." almondbreeze.com. http://www.almondbreeze.com/ (accessed June 9, 2015).

11. Centers for Disease Control and Prevention. "Data & Statistics." cdc.gov. www.cdc.gov/ncbddd/autism/data.html (accessed June 9, 2015).

12. Consumer Reports. "How Much Tuna Is Safe?" consumerreports.org. http://www.consumerreports.org/cro/magazine-archive/2011/january/food/mercury-in-tuna/how-much-tuna/index.htm (accessed June 9, 2015).

13. Daniels, SR, and Greer, FR. "Lipid Screening and Cardiovascular Health in Childhood." *Pediatrics* no. 1 (July 2008): 198–208.

14. Fitch, C, and Keim, KS. "Position of the Academy of Nutrition and Dietetics: use of nutritive and nonnutritive sweeteners." *Journal of the Academy of Nutrition and Dietetics* no. 8 (August 2012): 739–758.

15. Gidding, Samuel S., et al. "Dietary recommendations for children and adolescents: a guide for practitioners." *Pediatrics* no. 2 (February 2006): 544–559.

16. Gorski PA. "Toilet Training Guidelines: Clinicians—The Role of the Clinician in Toilet Training." *Pediatrics* no.6, Part 2(June 1999): 1364–66.

17. Harvard Medical School. "By the Way, Doctor: Children and Soy Milk." health.harvard.edu. http://www.health.harvard.edu/newsletters/Harvard_Health_Letter/2009/May/By-the-way-doctor-Children-and-soy-milk (accessed June 9, 2015).

18. Harvard School of Public Health. "Eggs and Heart Disease." hsph.harvard.edu. http://www.hsph.harvard.edu/nutritionsource/eggs/ (accessed June 9, 2015).

19. Harvard School of Public Health. "Artificial Sweeteners." hsph.harvard.edu. http://www.hsph.harvard.edu/nutritionsource/healthy-drinks/artificial-sweeteners/ (accessed June 9, 2015).

20. Hoffman, DR, and Boettcher, JA, et al. "Toward optimizing vision and cognition in term infants by dietary docosahexaenoic and arachidonic acid supplementation: a review of randomized controlled trials." *Prostaglandins, Leukotrienes and Essential Fatty Acids* no. 2 (August–September 2009): 151–158.

21. Hu, FB, Stampfer, MJ, and Rimm, EB, et al. "A prospective study of egg consumption and risk of cardiovascular disease in men and women." pubmed.gov. http://www.ncbi.nlm.nih.gov/pubmed/10217054?dopt=Citation (accessed June 9, 2015).

22. Iannelli, Vincent. "Is Fish Oil Right for Kids?" pediatrics.about.com. http://pediatrics.about.com/od/vitamins/a/Fish-Oil-Fish-Oil-Supplements-For-Kids.htm (accessed June 9, 2015).

23. Johns Hopkins Hospital, Jason Robertson, Nicole Shilkofski. *The Harriet Lane Handbook*, 17th edition. Philadelphia, PA: Elsevier Mosby, 2005.

24. Judd, RH. "Chronic Nonspecific Diarrhea." *Pediatrics in Review* no. 17 (November 1996): 379–384.

25. Mari-Bauset, S, and Mari-Sanchis, A, et al. "Evidence of the gluten-free and casein-free diet in autism spectrum disorders: a systemic review. " *J Child Neurol* no. 12 (December 2014): 1718.

26. Mead Johnson Nutrition. "Enfagrow Toddler Next Step Natural Milk Flavor." meadjohnson.com. http://www.meadjohnson.com/pediatrics/us-en/product-information/products/toddlers/enfagrow-toddler-next-step-natural-milk-flavor#nutrients-sup-sup (accessed June 9, 2015).

27. Meyenberg. "Whole Goat Milk Products." http://meyenberg.com/wp-content/uploads/QA-212-Nutritional-Info-Whole-Powdered-Milk.pdf (accessed January 8, 2016).

28. National Agricultural Library. http://ndb.nal.usda.gov/ (accessed June 9, 2015).

29. National Institute of Health. "Vitamin D: Fact Sheet for Health Professionals." ods.od.nih.gov. http://ods.od.nih.gov/factsheets/VitaminD-HealthProfessional/ (accessed June 9, 2015).

30. National Institute of Allergy and Infectious Diseases. "Guidelines for the Diagnosis and Management of Food Allergy in the United States." niaid.nih.gov. http://www.niaid.nih.gov/topics/foodallergy/clinical/Pages/default.aspx (accessed June 9, 2015).

31. Osborn, DA, Sinn, JK. "Probiotics in infants for prevention of allergic diseases and food hypersensitivity." *Cochrane Database Syst Review* no. 4 (October 2007).

32. Pan, A, and Sun, Q. "Red Meat Consumption and Mortality: Results from Two Prospective Cohort." *Archives of Internal Medicine* no. 7 (April 2012): 555–563.

33. Patisaul, HB, Jefferson W, "The pros and cons of phytoestrogen." *Frontiers in Neuroendocrinology* no. 4 (October 2010): 400–419.

34. Pennisi, CM, and Klein, LC. "Effectiveness of the gluten-free, casein free diet for children diagnosed with autism spectrum disorder: based on parental report." *Nutr Neurosci* no. 2 (March 2012): 85–91.

35. Pereira, MA, O'Reilly, E, and Augustsson, K, et al. "Dietary Fiber and Risk of Coronary Heart Disease: A Pooled Analysis of Cohort Studies." *Arch Intern Med* no. 4 (February 2004): 370–376.

36. Phillips, KM, and Carlsen, MH, et al. "Total antioxidant content of alternatives to refined sugar." *Journal of the American Dietetic Association* no. 1 (January 2009): 64–71.

37. Rong, Y, and Chen, L, et al. "Egg consumption and risk of coronary heart disease and stroke: dose-response meta-analysis of prospective cohort studies." *BMJ* no. 346 (January 2013): 1–13.

38. Rudolph, Abraham, Julien Hoffman, and Colin Rudolph. *Rudolph's Pediatrics, 20th edition.* Stamford, CT: Appleton & Lange, 1996.

39. Silk. "Vanilla Soy Milk." silk.com. http://silk.com/products/vanilla-soymilk (accessed June 9, 2015).

40. So Delicious Dairy Free. "Vanilla Coconut Milk Beverage." sodeliciousdairyfree.com. http://sodeliciousdairyfree.com/products/coconut-milk-beverages/vanilla (accessed June 9, 2015).

41. Taste the Dream. "Rice Dream Enriched Vanilla." tastethedream.com. http://www.tastethedream.com/products/product/1474/202.php (accessed June 9, 2015).

42. Texas Children's Hospital, Houston. *Texas Children's Hospital Pediatric Nutrition Reference Guide 10th edition.* Houston, Texas: Texas Children's Hospital, February 2014.

43. Thomas, DW, and Greer, FR. "Probiotics and Prebiotics in Pediatrics." *Pediatrics* no. 6 (December 2010): 1217–1231.

44. United States Department of Agriculture. "How many can I have?" choosemyplate.gov. http://www.choosemyplate.gov/weight-management-calories/calories/empty-calories-amount.html (accessed June 9, 2015).

45. United States Department of Agriculture. "Salt." choosemyplate.gov. http://www.choosemyplate.gov/preschoolers/daily-food-plans/about-salt.html (accessed June 9, 2015).

46. United States Department of Agriculture. "What are empty calories?" choosemyplate.gov. http://www.choosemyplate.gov/weight-management-calories/calories/empty-calories.html (accessed June 9, 2015).

47. United States Food and Drug Administration. "FDA Cuts Trans Fats in Processed Foods." http://www.fda.gov/ForConsumers/ConsumerUpdates/ucm372915.htm (Accessed June 9, 2015).

48. United States Food and Drug Administration. "Fish: What Pregnant Women and Parents Should Know." fda.gov. http://www.fda.gov/Food/FoodborneIllnessContaminants/Metals/ucm393070.htm (accessed June 9, 2015).

49. United States Food and Drug Administration. "National Nutrition Database." http://ndb.nal.usda.gov/udb/foods (accessed June 9, 2015).

50. Wagner, CL, and Greer, FR. "Prevention of Rickets and Vitamin D Deficiency in Infants, Children, and Adolescents." *Pediatrics* no. 5 (November 2008): 1142–1152.

51. Vanderhoof, JA. "Chronic Diarrhea." *Pediatrics in Review* no. 19 (December 1998): 418–422.

52. Weickert, MO, and Pfeiffer, AF. "Metabolic effects of dietary fiber consumption and prevention of diabetes." *The Journal of Nutrition* no. 3 (March 2008): 439–442.

53. Woosa, RK, and Thien, FC, et al. "Dietary marine fatty acids (fish oil) for asthma in adults and children." *Cochrane Database Syst Rev* no. 2 (April 2002).

Chapter Six: Common Medical Conditions and Additional Resources

1. Academy of Nutrition and Dietetics, Evidence Analysis Library. "Nutrition Celiac Disease Toolkit." andeal.org. http://andevidenceanalysislibrary.com (accessed June 9, 2015).

2. American Academy of Pediatrics. "Kids Need Fiber." http://www.healthychildren.org/English/healthy-living/nutrition/Pages/Kids-Need-Fiber-Heres-Why-and-How.aspx (accessed June 9, 2015)

3. American Academy of Pediatrics. *Pediatric Nutrition Handbook*, 6th Edition. Elk Grove Village, IL: 2008.

4. Berseth, CL. *Avery's Diseases of the Newborn, 7th ed*ition. Philadelphia: W. B. Saunders, 1998.

5. Gummyvites. "Fiber Gummy Bears." http://www.gummyvites.com/en/Lil-Critters/Products/Lil-Critters-Fiber-Gummy-Bears/Supplement-Facts (accessed January 11, 2016).

6. Harvard School of Public Health. "Fiber." http://www.hsph.harvard.edu/nutritionsource/carbohydrates/fiber/ (accessed June 9, 2015).

7. Mayo Clinic. "Chart of high-fiber foods." http://www.mayoclinic.org/healthy-living/nutrition-and-healthy-eating/in-depth/high-fiber-foods/art-20050948 (accessed June 9, 2015).

8. Metawellness. "Metamucil Original Coarse Powder." http://www.metawellness.com/en-us/products/fiber-powder/metamucil-original-coarse-powder (accessed January 11, 2016).

9. National Institute of Allergy and Infectious Diseases. "Guidelines for Diagnosis and Management of Food Allergy in the United States." niaid.nih.gov. http://www.niaid.nih.gov/topics/foodAllergy/clinical/Documents/FAGuidelinesExecSummary.pdf (accessed June 9, 2015).

10. Nelson, SP, and Chen, EH. "Prevalence of Symptoms of Gastroesophageal Reflux during Infancy." *Arch Pediatr Adolesc Med* no. 6 (June 1997): 569–572.

11. Nunes, Keith. "Mintel: Gluten free will hit $8.8 billion in sales in 2014." *Food Business News* (November 2014).

12. Tabbers, MM, and DiLorenzo, C. "Evaluation and Treatment of Functional Constipation in Infants and Children: Evidence-Based Recommendations from ESPGHAN and NASPGHAN." *Pediatrics* no. 2 (February 2014): 258–274.

13. Vandenplas, Y, and Rudolph, CD. "Pediatric Gastroesophageal Reflux Clinical Practice Guidelines: Joint Recommendations of the North American Society for Pediatric Gastroenterology, Hepatology, and Nutrition (NASPGHAN) and the European Society for Pediatric Gastroenterology, Hepatology, and Nutrition (ESPGHAN)." *JPGN* no. 49 (October 2009): 498–547.

14. Volta, U, and Bardell, MT, et al. "An Italian prospective multicenter survey on patients suspected of having non-celiac gluten sensitivity." *BMC Medicine* no. 12 (May 2014).

15. Wagner, CL, Greer, FR. American Academy of Pediatrics and the Section on Breastfeeding and Committee on Nutrition. "Prevention of Rickets and Vitamin D Deficiency in Infants, Children, and Adolescents" *Pediatrics* no 4. (November 2008) 1142–52.

Index

Copyright © 2016 by Anthony F. Porto, M.D. and Dina M. DiMaggio, M.D.
Cover photograph copyright © 2016 by Ashley Lima

All rights reserved.
Published in the United States by Ten Speed Press, an imprint of the Crown Publishing Group, a division of Penguin Random House LLC, New York.
www.crownpublishing.com
www.tenspeed.com

Ten Speed Press and the Ten Speed Press colophon are registered trademarks of Penguin Random House LLC.

Library of Congress Cataloging-in-Publication Data
Porto, Anthony.
 The pediatrician's guide to feeding babies and toddlers : practical answers to your questions on nutrition, starting solids, allergies, picky eating, and more / Anthony Porto, M.D. and Dina DiMaggio, M.D.
     pages cm
 Includes bibliographical references and index.
 1. Infants—Nutrition. 2. Children—Nutrition. 3. Food habits. I. Dimaggio, Dina Md. II. Title.
 RJ216.P66 2016
 618.92'02—dc23
                        2015031409

Trade Paperback ISBN: 978-1-60774-901-1
eBook ISBN: 978-1-60774-902-8

Printed in the United States of America

Design by Tatiana Pavlova
Illustrations by Betsy Stromberg

10 9 8 7 6 5 4 3 2 1

First Edition